A PLUME BOOK

THE GORGEOUSLY GREEN DIET

SOPHIE ULIANO is the author of the *New York Times* bestseller *Gorgeously Green*. An environmentalist since childhood, she has appeared as an eco-expert on many television shows, including *The Oprah Winfrey Show*, *The View*, *Good Morning America*, *iVillage Live*, and Discovery's *Planet Green*. She now has a national platform as a speaker and eco-expert. Her Web site, www.gorgeouslygreen.com, is a popular online community for like-minded women, featuring how-to videos, newsletters, monthly giveaways, and more. She lives in Los Angeles with her husband and daughter.

ALSO BY SOPHIE ULIANO

Gorgeously Green: 8 Simple Steps to an Earth-Friendly Life

THE
Gorgeously
GREEN DIET

SOPHIE ULIANO

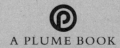

A PLUME BOOK

PLUME
Published by the Penguin Group

Penguin Group (USA) Inc., 375 Hudson Street, New York, New York 10014, U.S.A. • Penguin Group (Canada), 90 Eglinton Avenue East, Suite 700, Toronto, Ontario, Canada M4P 2Y3 (a division of Pearson Penguin Canada Inc.) • Penguin Books Ltd., 80 Strand, London WC2R 0RL, England • Penguin Ireland, 25 St. Stephen's Green, Dublin 2, Ireland (a division of Penguin Books Ltd.) • Penguin Group (Australia), 250 Camberwell Road, Camberwell, Victoria 3124, Australia (a division of Pearson Australia Group Pty. Ltd.) • Penguin Books Pvt. Ltd., 11 Community Centre, Panchsheel Park, New Delhi – 110 017, India • Penguin Group (NZ), 67 Apollo Drive, Rosedale, North Shore 0632, New Zealand (a division of Pearson New Zealand Ltd.) • Penguin Books (South Africa) (Pty.) Ltd., 24 Sturdee Avenue, Rosebank, Johannesburg 2196, South Africa

Penguin Books Ltd., Registered Offices: 80 Strand, London WC2R 0RL, England

Published by Plume, a member of Penguin Group (USA) Inc. Previously published in a Dutton edition.

First Plume Printing, January 2010
1 3 5 7 9 10 8 6 4 2

℗ REGISTERED TRADEMARK—MARCA REGISTRADA

The Library of Congress has catalogued the Dutton edition as follows:
Uliano, Sophie.
The gorgeously green diet : how to live lean and green / by Sophie Uliano.
p. cm.
ISBN 978-0-525-95115-5 (hc.)
ISBN 978-0-452-29591-9 (pbk.)
1. Sustainable living. 2. Natural foods. 3. Organic living. I. Title
GF78.U43 2009
640—dc22
2009006475

Printed in the United States of America
Original hardcover design by Spring Hoteling
Title page illustration by Robert Rodriguez
Exercise illustrations by Jaya Miceli

To my mother, Rachael, and my little treasure, Lola

CONTENTS

THE
Gorgeously
GREEN DIET

SECTION ONE
The Gorgeously Green Diet

CHAPTER ONE

Making a Difference

How many times do you wind up at the end of a day feeling burned out? Wishing someone else, for once, could plan, shop, and cook? How often have you drawn a blank when trying to figure out what on earth to have for lunch, never mind what you're going to cook for dinner? If you're time challenged and living on a tight budget, like many women, you've probably become bored and totally disillusioned with food, diets, and cooking. You know you should be preparing healthier meals, but what exactly does that mean? And how can you fit it into your already frazzled day? Many of us would love to be the perfect nontoxic mom/girlfriend with a washboard tummy and a gourmet organic dinner waiting, but reality hits. We're aching to do the right thing for ourselves and our planet, but how exactly do we go about this?

Although I try my best to lead a Gorgeously Green life, it's easy to become stressed, tired, and frustrated. There are days when I wind up galloping through my day, grabbing sugar-laden snacks, barely chewing my food, desperate to get the next thing ticked off my to-do list. I realize that on these rushed days, I'm only half living my life because I'm missing the very tastes and textures, the details that should be bringing me joy. It's become my passion and mission to change this, because ultimately I always want my eating choices to be the best they can be. I also want to be bursting with sparkling energy. I want to celebrate my love of great food with every mouthful I take.

Food is the source of life, and yet, for the most part, we have totally lost that connection. Zipping through the grocery store, throwing garish convenience packets into our cart, has become a deadening experience. Not to mention our confusion about what we should and shouldn't be eating and, most notably, what, oh horror of horrors, will make us chubby. The irony is that, in our attempt to do the right thing, we are unwittingly eating the very foods that are making us fat, tired, and sick.

Unless the food you buy is minimally processed and packaged, unless it's locally produced and organic—in short, unless its Gorgeously Green—it's likely to be lacking in vitamins and loaded with toxins that could inhibit metabolism and lead to obesity. Convenience food might taste good for a few seconds, but the price we have to pay in terms of feeling worn-out, sluggish, and empty is just not worth it.

Low-quality food is overstressing the planet and making it dangerously sick, too: Millions of pounds of pesticides and herbicides leach into our soil and dwindling clean water supplies, and our landfills are maxed out with obscene amounts of unnecessary food packaging. What we do to the planet, we do to ourselves, and vice versa. It's high time that we put our health first so that we can heal our worn-out bodies and our depleted planet.

Now is the moment for change, and I have a great deal of hope that we can, one day at a time, take small steps to bring our health, energy, and even our skinny jeans back, while helping to make this planet habitable for our children's children. How we eat affects every day of our life and is the legacy we leave behind.

The other day, I was compelled to slow down as I found myself in the ramshackle kitchen of Bill Spencer on his organic farm in San Luis Obispo, California. I had dropped in on him, unannounced, as I had heard that he grew the most delicious heirloom tomatoes on earth. Bill was out on his tractor but assured me that he could chat when he was done with the field if I didn't mind watching him cook, for it was baking day. I stood waiting in his sunny living room, looking out onto grapevines, olive trees, and apple orchards beyond. Time suddenly stood still, and all I could hear were the baby lambs bleating in his front yard and the woodpeckers stashing acorns in the massive oak tree outside.

Later, as Bill and I chatted, the aroma of his sourdough loaf, baking in the tiny oven, wafted over us, cozy and healing. We later ate it, still warm and slathered in soft, yellow butter. He handed me a slice of his award-winning Golden Girl tomato. I savored each mouthful—it would have been rude not to, for each bite brought different subtle tastes of sweet summer bliss. I know that I can't have a Farmer Bill experience very often in my crazy, challenged-mommy lifestyle, but I do acknowledge that I have to slow down more often.

Part of the problem is that eating low-quality food makes us want to rush. I sat down to eat a salad at the airport recently, and as much as I tried, I couldn't even nibble at the thick, cold slab of pale tomato perched atop a chunk of uninviting iceberg lettuce. No wonder people wolf this sort of thing down, I thought, as I guiltily shoved the plastic container into the trash. I am fortunate enough to love salads, but I need taste and texture—dark green leaves bursting with nutrition, and sweet, fruity tomatoes drizzled in olive oil and sprinkled with herbs.

Strawberries say it all: When I was young, they were a precious treat that was available only in season and so around for just a couple of months a year. I remember sitting on our doorstep with a bowl of freshly picked berries still warm from the sun. Covered in thick, clotted cream and crunchy brown sugar, each bite was a delectable taste of creamy caramel, followed by thick, juicy sweetness. In comparison, if I bite into a nonorganic, grocery store strawberry in December, its watery texture and bitter tang completely fail to satisfy and leave me craving something sweet. To add insult to injury, those seemingly innocent strawberries are the most heavily sprayed fruit crop on the planet, so I probably got a good dose of pesticide residue. So did the waterways surrounding the fields, and so did everyone drinking water.

CHAPTER TWO

Your Eco-Impact

One of the most powerful ways you can make a difference is by changing your diet. This is because the way you eat involves so many different choices that directly affect the health of our planet. What is your eco-impact? Do your daily actions regarding food have a positive or a negative impact on the environment? These are questions I ask myself every day because the most powerful legacy I can leave behind is to have lived with the lightest footprint possible. It's unachievable to be the *perfect* Green Girl; however, I can take simple, powerful steps toward this end: You vote with your dollars, and each day you make hundreds of choices. What to buy? Where to buy it? How to cook it? The list goes on and on—so why not make every single one of these choices have a positive rather than a negative impact on the environment?

The Gorgeously Green Diet takes the middle road. It's all about balance. I'm not advocating that from now on you should shop only at expensive health food stores and buy *everything* organic. On the contrary, this diet is about taking small, everyday steps that make sense for your busy and budget-challenged lives. For many, the closest we'll ever get to an organic farm is a picture in a magazine. We can, however, bring elements of that farm to our own backyards and window boxes by planting heirloom tomatoes and baby salad leaves, even a little olive tree. Moreover, we can allow those glossy pictures to remind us that farming methods still exist that value quality over quantity and health over profit.

My mission is to create outrageously delicious food with the freshest ingredients possible at the lowest price. I haven't got time to fiddle around in my kitchen for hours, so part of my mission also is to create meals that are speedy and fun. It can be thrilling to throw together a beautiful, organic soup in twenty minutes (to feed a family of four), rather than to open a couple of cans. The Gorgeously Green Diet is all about creating mouthwatering and inexpensive meals.

Eating the Gorgeously Green way is simply a win/win situation because it's:

Better for your health
Better for your pocketbook
Better for maintaining your ideal weight

Here are just a few ways in which we can lighten our footprint:

If every American bought just one minimally packaged item out of every ten food purchases, the waste eliminated from landfills each year would be enough to cover New York City's Central Park with a twenty-seven-foot-high layer of garbage.

If every American shifted just *one* day per week's food calories from red meat and dairy to chicken, fish, eggs, and vegetables, the reduction in greenhouse gas emissions would be equivalent to 760 miles of driving per year. If they shifted just *one* day a week's food calories from red meat to fruits and veggies, that would be equivalent to 1,160 miles of driving, and if they became vegetarian, the impact of their driving would be entirely negated!

If every American used just one reusable tote for each shopping trip, we could save more than 60,000 trees.

As you can see, small changes can wind up making a big difference. We can all cut out red meat for just one day a week, and by doing so we invest in our health, our planet, and our savings accounts. When hearing these statistics, my sister-in-law, Kay, decided to cut red meat from her diet completely. "If it's that easy to make such a difference," she said, "I'll do it." She's also thrilled that she's cutting her grocery bills down considerably and has even lost weight.

DIETS

Overwhelmed and confused, many of us have spent years on a feast-or-famine yo-yo diet. We've lost our love of food and our connection to its source. We've unwittingly abused our bodies, our souls, and our planet. Reaching for a zero-fat, zero-carb packet containing a tasteless and empty promise is downright depressing. It's time to get back to savoring the startling crunch of a fresh apple or the unbelievable comfort of a bowl of buttery mashed potatoes. When is the last time you bit into a coffee bean just because, or sank your hand into a bowl of polished, uncooked rice? When is the last time you popped a square of dark, velvety chocolate into your mouth and let it melt, really slowly, as you let your thoughts wander? Foods like this aren't what make us fat. It's how we eat them. This is what is killing us, and the planet.

REAL FOOD

The Gorgeously Green Diet is primarily about rediscovering the joys of eating real, whole foods so you can become the healthiest Green Girl imaginable.

I remember standing gossiping over a steaming mug of tea with my great friend Nancy in her impossibly tidy, newly tricked-out kitchen. It's one of those kitchens that boasts a shiny Viking range that (a) you wish you owned and (b) you know has *never* been cooked on. Suddenly her Jessica Alba lookalike teenage daughter, Zoe, rushed in to "grab a bite" before going out for the evening. Her dinner amounted to a "Stab-Stab." I call frozen convenience meals Stab-Stabs because you basically whip it out of the freezer, stab it twice with a fork, and stuff it into the microwave. Standing in her tiny denim shorts and furry sheepskin boots, Zoe cooked her Stab-Stab on high for two minutes, ripped off the plastic cover, and stood eating it with a fork while checking her text messages. Her mother, whom I adore, didn't bat an eyelash. I try not to judge, because before I had my daughter Lola, I was all about "I'll never let my baby eat sugar or have plastic toys, etc.," and then after, cut to enough sugar on a weekend to make Willy Wonka's hair stand on end. However, I did watch with horror while a teenager, whose body is still critically developing, was not even eating real food. The Stab-Stab in question was a diet mac and cheese. Through my research, I know the brand well and shudder to think what is going into her system: genetically modified wheat, hormone-riddled milk and cheese, and a bunch of chemicals and preservatives. I don't call that real food. It's an imitation of real food that could wind up making this beautiful girl unhappy and obese in years to come if she eats enough of it. This kind of food is also catastrophic for the environment: The pesticides and herbicides that are typically used to grow the wheat devastate the soil and water. Combined with the packaging, they use an enormous amount of polluting petrochemicals and energy. I'm sure if this highly intelligent girl really understood the eco-impact of that one seemingly innocent meal, she'd change her ways pretty fast.

Convenience food is where the food industry makes all of its money. It's the one area where they can keep marking up the price and lowering the quality. You are paying primarily for the packaging and advertising: Almost a quarter of every food dollar you spend goes to marketing. Yes—you're paying for commercials that encourage you and your kids to eat extremely bad-quality food. Another quarter of every food dollar you spend goes on that extremely difficult-to-open package. If you care about the planet at all, which I assume you do because you are reading this book, the packaging that you eventually managed to rip off is winging its way to an overstuffed landfill as you read.

The big food companies also know our every move. They study our lifestyles down to the exact number of minutes we spend in our kitchens on a daily basis. They rub their hands together with glee as they know that the average time spent preparing food in a kitchen is soon to be as little as five minutes. That's a few more Caribbean vacations for them, because we'll need more and more fake food. Thrilled, they can go back to their laboratories and dream up the next vitamin/probiotic-infused, low-fat Pop-Tart that cooks in just fifteen seconds. Maybe by then we'll have a microwave/computer/iPhone gadget so we can check our messages while the tart gets blasted—why not save fifteen precious seconds if we can?

I resolutely refuse to become one of those food company "statistics"—and I encourage you to do the same. Let's outwit them. Let's get back into our kitchens and start preparing the sort of food we dream about. It's so much easier than you think.

POTS OF GOLD

The other industry that is making a mockery of us is the diet food/supplement industry. These clever guys know that we all want to get thin without doing the obvious: eating less and exercising more. They know that we are looking for an easier, softer way. They know we want a miracle pill or food that will make us shrink down like Alice in Wonderland without changing one of our miserable habits. They also know that we'll pay through the roof for this miracle cure. We give these dudes our money and our power and it never, ever works.

Evolution has programmed us to eat until we are beyond full, because in the days of scarcity when our ancestors were running around in fur skirts, hunting for berries and roots, calories were the thing. You had to find your sources of energy or your muscles would stop functioning and you'd basically drop dead. In times of abundance, when they were able to take down a huge hairy boar, for instance, their bodies evolved to eat and store more food than they needed so that they'd survive times of scarcity, which was every other day. They also evolved a liking for sweet and fatty things, since animal fat and sugar provided the most energy for hunting. Fast-forward to modern times and we still have the same biology as our ancestors, the same biochemical processes that tell us when and what we need to eat, yet we have completely different lifestyles. Instead of hunting for eight hours a day, we sit at a desk or computer. Most of us don't know the meaning of scarcity, and we eat chips, sodas, and frozen meals that are packed with more than double the amount of calories of fresh, whole foods. Wow—we are in deep trouble. No wonder 50 percent of America is now grossly overweight and childhood obesity is an epidemic.

CONVENIENCE/FAST FOODS VERSUS WHOLE/FRESH FOODS

An apple with 1 tablespoon almond butter = 176 calories
A convenience store blueberry muffin = 310 calories

The great news is that we have a choice. We can take back our power from the $5 billion-a-year diet industry and from the gazillion-dollar-a-year food industry, and we can start making choices that defy our genetics and sedentary lifestyles.

CHAPTER THREE

See It

The first step in becoming empowered and gorgeous is to visualize how you would like your life to be. What are the things you want to change?

I wanted to become as healthy as I could and I wanted as many of my food choices to be as eco-friendly as possible. I chose health over thin because healthy is sexy, whereas *too* thin can be unattractive. Ask any man! Women's bodies are supposed to be curvaceous and soft. Doesn't it make you shudder to see photographs of various celebrities with eating disorders? Beautiful young girls turn into wiry, old-looking women in a matter of months. Unless you are under twenty, your body isn't supposed to look like a teenager's. It's also really annoying that women over a certain age, when they lose a lot of weight suddenly, can look twice their age—we need fat on our faces to keep the bloom of youth, and that's the first area that goes (in my case, my bust, too). So back to healthy=sexy. We all have different body shapes, which are largely determined by our genetics, but we can do an awful lot with the cards we've been dealt. So my intention and vision is to see myself as vibrant, healthy, and glowing, and I know that if I am all of the above, I will be the exact weight I am supposed to be. It's all about finding a natural balance, and this is what the Gorgeously Green Diet will help you do.

If you need to lose weight for your health and happiness, I promise you will. If you need to gain a few pounds (I know, most people are furious to think that any such woman exists!), you will, too. Most important, if you really care about your health *and* the health of the planet, the Gorgeously Green Diet will help you to attain your vision.

VISUALIZATION EXERCISE

1. Identify what you want: What does it look like and feel like? (E.g., I want to feel healthier, stronger, and more connected to the earth.)
2. Where in your life do you currently have some of this? (E.g., When I make time to do yoga and on the days I commit to buying only healthy food.)
3. What are the obstacles in my life that keep me from being able to attain my vision? (E.g., I don't have time for yoga/exercise every day. I can't always afford to buy healthy food. I'm always in a rush.)
4. What are the different choices I can make to help me attain my vision? (E.g., I can put aside just ten minutes a day for yoga. I can make a list of only the most important foods to buy organic. I can take a daily walk as a meditation to reflect on what is great about my life.)

DESERVING

Do you believe that you are worth really taking care of? Do you deserve the best? Many of us are so caught up in taking care of everyone else that we've put ourselves last on the list. This is a dangerous situation because if your health suffers, then everyone else will suffer. Far from being selfish, taking great care of yourself will pay huge dividends to everyone around you. Only when your batteries are fully charged, only when you are sparkling with energy, can you be a gift to everyone in your life. Taking the time to follow a healthy, nutritious diet, to exercise, and to create a moment of stillness daily, where you acknowledge your vital, life-sustaining source, deep within, are necessary components to becoming the best you can be and living your life beautifully.

DON'T WORRY

If the thought of a filet mignon, a tuna melt, or a cheese pizza makes your mouth water, don't worry, because you will still be able to eat what you love. The secret is to value quality over quantity and to have a little bit of anything that you fancy.

The key to moderation obviously is portion size, and it's useful to remind ourselves that portion sizes have almost doubled since the 1970s: Dinner plates are bigger; chairs and beds are bigger and sturdier to accommodate our enormous bodies; bagels, cookies, bags of chips, and buckets of soda have more than doubled in size. And yet our lifestyles have become smaller. If you locked an animal in a small space, denied it much exercise, and yet doubled its caloric intake, you'd be accused of cruelty. I remember an old lady who used to live near us when I was little, and she overfed her spaniel (dogs that are supposed to be lean and active) to the point that it had trouble walking, let alone running. We were appalled, and yet now we are beginning to punish ourselves in the same way.

I took my small daughter, Lola, to a restaurant that I didn't want to go to, but she had been begging because she had heard that they served Shirley Temple cocktails for little girls, decorated with umbrellas and flowers. She had earned a treat or, to be perfectly honest, I think I was bribing her to tidy her room, so we took our seats and ordered the requisite drink—a terrifying pink globe filled with all the things that Mommy hates: dye, high-fructose corn syrup, artificial flavors, the lot. I asked her if it was good, praying she would say "not really," but, as she sucked away at the straw, her eyes grew as big as saucers. "It's soooooo good, Mommy," she gasped, before her lips clamped firmly around the nonrecyclable straw again. But what really put me off the whole adventure were the gargantuan portions floating past us. I am not exaggerating to say that one piled-high bowl of seafood pasta or Chinese chicken salad could have easily satisfied a family of four. Every now and again the waitress would come by and ask if the diner was "still working on it." I really dislike the term *working* on it, for it implies that eating is laborious and not pleasurable. However, in this restaurant, I would hazard to say that it was an absolute labor of love to finish the entire portion, and a couple of women were clearly trying their best.

So how do we go back to how we used to be thirty or so years ago when portions were half the size they are today? How do we do this without feeling the pinch, without feeling that we are denying—even starving—ourselves? It's simple: You cut your portion size down, and after seven to ten days, your stomach will adjust and you will feel full with half the amount. Don't forget that eating whole foods will also help you to feel satisfied. Forget every bit of weight-loss advice you've ever been given and just put back a third or half of what you would normally eat. If you are dealing with an enormous muffin or bagel, cut it in two and wrap up the remainder for tomorrow. If you are used to boil-

TIPS FOR CUTTING DOWN YOUR PORTION SIZES

- Use salad plates instead of dinner plates.
- Slow down and take time to experience the different tastes, colors, and textures of all the foods on your plate.
- Put your fork down between bites.
- Chew each mouthful thoroughly, savoring each and every bite.
- Take a ten-minute break before reaching for a second helping. You may find that you are actually pretty full. We tend to plow so quickly through our food that we stop listening to our internal cues.
- Stop eating when you are 80 percent full. If that's hard for you to gauge, put down your fork before your stomach feels completely full and wait for five minutes before you pick it up again.

ing a whole fourteen-ounce packet of pasta for two people (that was me), then take out only half. If you order or make a sandwich for your lunch, make it with one slice of bread so you effectively have half a sandwich. Use your salad plates for your main course instead of the oversize dinner plate. Whether or not you want to lose weight, it's a good idea to radically cut down, because they say that lean people live much longer. And we need you around for the duration, because you are going to inspire women for years to come with your Gorgeously Green beauty and vitality. Plus, smaller portions mean less money spent—you'll be able to stretch your food budget much further.

There's one more plus in cutting back portion size—your wallet! Yes, you will save a lot of money by sticking to the serving-size suggestion on the box of pasta or splitting an eight-ounce steak in half—especially if you have a big family. I am well aware that there are certain family members who will rail against you, but persist until they get used to it. The key is to sneak it a bit smaller every day so they won't really notice. Another great idea is to get smaller dinner plates from flea markets. I have a 1950s restaurant line of dinnerware that I purchased from a flea market years ago. I never used the dinner plates because they seemed too small; however, they've now been dusted off and reinstituted as our regular daily plates, so no one feels too deprived by the smaller portions.

At a restaurant, where portion sizes are often absurdly enormous, consider:

- Ordering two appetizers instead of an appetizer and an entrée
- Sharing an entrée with your partner or friend
- Asking for a half (appetizer-size) portion of your chosen entrée
- Asking for half of your entrée to be packaged up for you to take home★

★ Ask for a "doggie bag" only if you know you will eat the leftovers the next day. We often ask for this packaging because we feel guilty wasting the food; however, you're better off getting a smaller portion in the first place.

STARVING?

You will not go hungry on this diet. On the contrary, you will feel more satisfied than you ever have. The key to losing weight is being satisfied. You will never stick to an eating plan that demands that you go hungry—of course not! This is why so many low-fat foods are counterproductive—you will feel hungry, really hungry, a couple of hours after eating them because you haven't had a dose of the healthy fats that make you feel full. The other foods that guarantee to make you feel full although you're starving are refined carbs: A bagel or corn muffin will send your blood sugar sky-high and signal the pancreas to pump out insulin to bring it back down. The problem is that it often comes crashing down a couple of hours later, making you run to the coffee shop or the fridge for a sugary drink or a snack—anything to pull you through until your next meal. You can still enjoy delicious breads and pastries, but we're going to make sure that all the ingredients are recognizable and that they are made with organic, whole grains, which will *slowly* release the sugar into your bloodstream, giving your poor old pancreas a break!

Growing up in England involved eating a lot of saturated fat (yummy butter, cream, and cheese). Actually, my favorite dessert as a little girl was bizarrely named "Spotted Dick" and was made of suet (flour and lard) and raisins (the spots)—it was always served with copious amounts of custard or heavy cream. I ate all this to my heart's content and yet was nicknamed "Shrimp" at school because I was so tiny and thin. As I became more aware of nutrition and not wanting to pack on the pounds as a paranoid twenty-something, I turned my back on my deliciously fatty upbringing. I spent years avoiding fatty fats, wrongly thinking that they were the sole cause of hideous cellulite. My brother didn't have to worry about a summer vacation skimpy bikini, so he kept eating Mom's delicious fatty offerings and never put on a single pound. Conversely, my weight went up and down with each new food fad I came across. Like many women, I've been swayed by the winds of virtually every media diet craze that ever was.

As a theater actress in London, I always felt the pressure to be pencil thin. So the struggle to find the miracle diet was constant. Then something happened that changed the way I ate forever: I got a job working for a year in one of England's legendary regional theaters. I wasn't thrilled, however, that I was going to have to move up to a little town near the misty moors of Yorkshire in the chilly North, the birthplace of Yorkshire pudding, a sort of pancake batter fried in lard. There wasn't a health shop or diet food in sight, and so I just threw in the towel and ate like a local: fish and chips, roast chicken, vegetables slathered in butter, and freshly picked blackberries with whipped cream. Oddly enough, I felt fantastic and, six months later, found that I had actually lost ten pounds! My skin was better and my mood swings leveled out. Most important, I rediscovered the joy of eating really yummy food and realized that it was the carbs and sugars, not the fat, that had made my weight fluctuate so much. Fifteen years later, I'm still here to tell the tale and have pretty much maintained a perfect weight while eating loads of healthy fats. As I have explored the diets of many traditional cultures all over the world, I have discovered that the healthiest people do not eat diet, health, or convenience foods. Traditional diets tend to favor healthy fats, loads of vegetables, and a little meat and dairy. So if you, too, want to be a happy, satisfied girl with a relatively flat tummy, read on.

THE PROMISE

Having got so caught up in the calorie/carb/fat paranoia, we've lost our ability to savor unadulterated moments of sweet-tasting ecstasy. I promise to bring all this back to you, served on a guiltless platter, and show you how to cook the best meal you've ever tasted—the kicker being that it won't harm you, the planet, or your budget. I will show you how to become more aware each and every day, so that you can give yourself and your family the very best that nature has to offer. I will show you how easy it is to lose the weight and the waste in your life without having to compromise in the pleasure department. I will show you how to find balance in an eating plan that you can customize according to the kind of Green Girl you really are.

There is never a quick fix to anything that is worthwhile. The good things in life are slow and require a bit of patience—whether it's the fermenting of grapes to create an exceptional bottle of wine or the rising of dough for your warm, crispy baguette. It's the same with a diet. Quick-fix diets—lose thirty pounds in thirty days—*never* last and always compromise your health on some level. The Gorgeously Green Diet is a slow diet but one that is sustainable. It's unlikely that after fourteen days, you'll spring up one morning to find that your body is a dead ringer for Victoria Beckham's or Kelly Ripa's. I will not make unrealistic and empty promises to you. I am more concerned that you will change your diet to a way of eating that will gradually, slowly transform your body, your beliefs, your enjoyment of food, and your impact on the planet and will last forever.

I have been eating like this for many years now, and I'm in better health than ever. I never weigh myself, for the same jeans fit today that fit five years ago. I am no longer willing to pay the price for eating cheap, low-quality food. I absolutely am what I eat, and because I choose not to walk around full of toxic residues and hormone-disrupting chemicals, I have decided to switch to eating only the foods that will help save my health and the health of the planet. As a result, I am strong, vibrant, and full of energy even on a day when I have chaos and a whining child in tow. I try to enjoy each and every morsel that I put into my mouth, knowing that it is beautiful "real" food—the best that nature has to offer—and that every choice I make will help lighten my impact on this still-gorgeous planet.

SECTION TWO
Gorgeously Green Diet Plans

CHAPTER FOUR

One Size Doesn't Fit All

CUSTOMIZE YOUR PLAN

The mistake with many diets is that they assume we're all at home all day long and have the time to fiddle around cooking fancy low-fat lunch entrées. Given the fact that almost 60 percent of women in America who are over the age of sixteen work, and that 75 percent of these women work in full-time office jobs, it only makes sense to create a diet that will work brilliantly for the working office girl, too. I provide an Office Girl option (OG) for every day.

We also live in different areas and have different incomes, time challenges, food preferences, children issues—the list goes on. So take a good look at the "Shades of Green" options below and see where you fit in.

SHADES OF GREEN

The other day a friend, Lena, confessed to me that she wasn't really very Green. After the confession, she held her breath as though I was about to start berating her! I asked her what she meant, and she explained that she eats totally unhealthy meals and even uses spray-on butter for convenience, and, she said, almost crying, "I can't stop using paper towels and Ziploc bags, I just can't, but I want to lose weight and get healthier and I do care about the polar bears drowning, I do!" I assured Lena that she wouldn't have to give up anything she didn't want to and that being Gorgeously Green is about making simple changes that work for you.

You absolutely don't need to give up every guilty pleasure, and for some of us, the eco-changes need to be baby steps at first. I realized after talking to Lena that I had to put my Shading System in place for this diet because we are all at different stages along the green path. While some of my friends are solar-backpack-wearing vegans, others are spray-butter girls like Lena. I want this diet to work for all of you, so pick your shade.

LIGHT GREEN

You're interested in becoming a little more eco-friendly; however, you're not willing to go over the top! You're afraid that many of the foods that you really love may be deemed too unhealthy for a Green Diet, but you want to do the right thing. Paper towels and napkins and your beloved microwave are part of the landscape of your kitchen and you can never remember which plastic numbers are recyclable and which are not. You're freaked out about global warming and pollution but not quite enough to give up getting your whites white with some good old chlorine bleach. You feel horribly guilty each time you walk out of the store with a gazillion plastic bags, but the two canvas totes you were given somehow got left behind in the laundry room. Once they made it as far as the trunk of your car but never made it out.

You're used to shopping at regular grocery stores and delis and you often eat in restaurants that couldn't, even on a good day, be described as earth friendly. You also like eating fast food and convenience food—it's what works for your time-challenged life. You've tried a few diets but none of them seemed to stick because extremes don't work for the kind of girl that you are. You want to start introducing some organic foods into your diet and you are attracted to living a greener life. However, you're on a very tight budget and/or have a lot of mouths to feed. Your beautiful shade is LIGHT GREEN.

BRIGHT GREEN

You desperately want to be more eco-friendly. You're ready to jump in and find out exactly what you need to do to ensure a healthier future for your children. You carry a reusable water bottle, know your "safe" plastics, recycle your paper and glass, but have yet to visit your local hazardous waste unit with your used batteries and curly, energy-saving lightbulbs. You've turned down your thermostat and switched to non-toxic cleaners, but you still buy gossip magazines and diet soda. You'll consider growing tomatoes this summer, but you've got grave misgivings about composting—especially with worms! You're ready and willing to make some dramatic changes in your diet and lifestyle if it means you will be healthier and happier.

In an ideal world, you would love to eat organically all the time, but it's not always possible, due to cost and availability. You are ready to go the extra mile for the sake of the planet, but you're not giving up your paper towels or your bagged salad yet. You may also have to contend with partners/families who are stubbornly clinging to unhealthy eating habits and who are in total denial about the state of the environment. You may have your work cut out for you. You are a vibrant BRIGHT GREEN.

DEEP GREEN

You're a Greenie through and through. You're perhaps vegetarian or vegan, or you eat *only* the most humanely reared, pasture-finished meat you can find. You wear your green on your feet, too, eschewing leather shoes and favoring hemp pumps with car-tire soles instead. You'll stop short of nothing that could lessen your already light eco-impact: backyard hens, heirloom carrots, even a compost toilet—your Green To Do List is growing by the minute. You'll step out of your comfort zone if need be and cycle to the barbeque, a veggie burger in your solar backpack, as you try not to judge your gas-guzzling, burger-eating friends. You live your deepest values, but you wouldn't mind a few tips to help take you to the next level and make your diet more practical, affordable, and fun.

You get a bit tired of the same old dishes and recipes, and you, like everyone else, would love to be a little healthier and a little lighter. You've found there are cost, convenience, and boredom issues with the way you want to eat, so you're on the lookout for a few helpful hints to make eating an utter delight. You are a delectable DEEP GREEN.

PICK YOUR SHADE

Time to choose which shade you most identify with. You may find that you cross over, in that you identify with aspects of two different shades. If this is the case, I suggest you pick the lighter one to start with. A friend of mine, Julia, identified with much of the Deep Green description, yet she started with the Bright Green eating plan, knowing she could graduate and move on.

The shades are not in order of virtuousness. If you are Light Green, you are not in the remedial group. It's simply about picking a plan that's a good fit for your lifestyle.

The diet plans last for fourteen days. I recommend you stick to the diet for at least thirty days. For the second fourteen days, repeat your plan but substitute with any recipes that take your fancy from the back of the book. I have provided more than one hundred delicious dishes for you to try.

Remember the Gorgeously Green Diet is a lifestyle change that includes a balanced eating and exercise plan. It's designed to be sustainable by being a way of eating you'll want to continue. Unlike many other diets, this one won't make you feel like you're "on a diet," because you get to eat normally. You also won't need to prepare separate meals for yourself and your family. This diet is a gift for all of you and will work whether you live alone or are a mother of five.

> The biggest-ever study on organic food was funded by the European Union. The four-year study found that organic produce contains 40 percent more antioxidants than nonorganic, and organic milk contains 60 percent more nutrients than nonorganic.

CHAPTER FIVE

Eating Plan Primer

Before you start your eating plan, take a look at the following recommendations. Although I'm going to suggest that you avoid many of the usual suspects like sodas, refined flours, and sugars, I'm not a food Nazi—rather, I'm a fervent believer in trying to eat in the healthiest way possible for most of the time and then allowing yourself to have regular and delicious treats, even if a bit of white flour or sugar creeps in. If you have built your system up to be strong and balanced, it will be able to cope with a few transgressions.

You'll find many of the following foods in the eating plan, so make sure you are familiar with all of them before you start.

There are so many questions when it comes to eco-friendly food, and sometimes the confusion and cost can be a turnoff. In the following list of foods, I have attempted to give you the whole picture of each given food, in the hope that you can make a more informed decision when you start shopping.

You may have friends and family who won't even consider buying healthier food because they are so set in their ways. One of their standard lines of attack is: "I've been eating like this for my whole life and it hasn't killed me yet!" I believe *yet* is the key word here even though there are always exceptions to the rule. Just as there's always that vigorous old crone puffing away on unfiltered cigarettes and boasting that she's "as fit as a fiddle," there may be a few of us as robust, but most of us aren't. Although eating one pesticide-laced strawberry may not make you sick, eating these toxins cumulatively over a long period of time can seriously harm you. We only need to look around at the escalating cancer and heart-disease statistics to be convinced.

IS SHOPPING ONLINE
ECO-FRIENDLY?

Each minute spent driving to the mall uses more than ten times the energy of a minute spent shopping online (when choosing ground shipping).

According to Joseph J. Romm, author and executive director of the Center for Energy and Climate Solutions, shipping ten pounds of packages by overnight air (the most intensive energy delivery mode) still used 40 percent less fuel than driving round-trip to the mall or grocery store. Ground shipping by truck uses only one-tenth the energy of driving yourself. So shopping online is eco-friendly, provided you don't pick the overnight-air option.

You may need to shop online for some of the recommended items, but keep in mind that shopping online has a lighter eco-impact than going to the store.

ECO-FRIENDLY FOOD

Eco-friendly food is more expensive; however, it's cheaper in the long run because you will save on health care bills later in life. Each time you weigh the pros and cons of a particular food, or agonize about whether or not to buy the organic version, just think about your precious health. I'd rather hold off buying a new television or the latest cell phone in favor of feeding my family on food that will keep us in good shape. We are what we eat.

We are used to eating cheap food in the United States because the massive industrial food system has managed to produce food on a gargantuan scale. The hidden costs of this food are safety, health, security, and environmental devastation. How much are you willing to pay to be sure that your ground beef won't poison you? How much are you willing to pay to ensure that your breads and crackers won't make you obese? How much are you willing to pay to ensure that you will always have a supply of good, fresh food? How much are you willing to pay for clean air, food, and water? These are the questions that we need to start asking ourselves when we panic over food prices.

The more expensive sustainable/organic foods that we see in the market reflect the true cost of the food. You don't get a piece of beautiful meat or a pesticide-free tomato without a lot of care and labor going into its production. The U.S. food system as we know it is beginning to break down: Outbreaks of *E. coli and Salmonella* food poisoning are becoming more commonplace, resulting in giant recalls of meat and dairy. Monoculture industrial farming (one crop only) is beginning to yield less food as the soil becomes devoid of nutrients through overuse of chemicals. Things have to change, and the challenge we are going to face is how to feed the hungry when those food systems become even worse. It's a romantic ideal to think that small-scale organic farming could even attempt to feed the hungry masses. However, these sustainable food producers serve as a model on which to build.

The Gorgeously Green Diet is more about making practical daily choices that everyone can afford than about joining an elite crowd who doesn't think twice about carting home boxes of organically prepared food in their plug-in hybrids. The most powerful signal you can send to the giant food industry is that you are less interested in processed pre-prepared foods because you have decided to cook at home three or four nights a week. This is real eco-friendly food—it's eco-nomical, too!

> **BEEFY FACTS**
> - Adopting a vegan diet actually does more to reduce harmful greenhouse gas emissions than driving a hybrid car.
> - You could drive a small car twenty miles on the energy required to produce a singe hamburger.
> - Every minute of every day, a land area equivalent to seven football fields is destroyed in the Amazon Basin for hamburger meat.

WHAT ABOUT MEAT?

Meat is a hugely contentious issue because many environmentalists think we should give meat up altogether. However, eating meat is deeply ingrained in our culture, and therefore it is really tough for many people to even consider cutting down. Although I don't recommend going from carnivore to full-on vegan in one fell swoop, I do recommend cutting back your meat consumption, especially beef. It will also save you a considerable amount of money.

HOW MUCH MEAT?

How much meat should we eat to be Gorgeously Green? Is it greener to use our land to grow vegetables or raise cattle? The answer is quite surprising. A Cornell University study in 2007 showed that a diet containing about *two* ounces of daily meat protein, as opposed to a vegan diet, was the most efficient in terms of land use. To get a visual, a deck of cards is about three to four ounces, so we're talking about a portion approximately the size of my daughter's mini iPod. I realized with horror that the sandwich I had purchased the other day at the deli contained at least three iPods' worth of sliced turkey. How did we get used to eating so much meat? My husband thought I was joking when I served him an iPod-size portion of chicken breast. "No, I'm not joking," I replied. "So, help yourself to more vegetables!" He wasn't thrilled, that is, not until a few weeks later, when he discovered to his amazement that his pants, which had hitherto been a little on the snug side, were literally hanging off him.

Dr. Rajendra Pachauri, chair of the UN Intergovernmental Panel on Climate Change, advocates giving up meat for at least one day a week initially and decreasing it from there. The UN's Food and Agricultural Organization has estimated that meat production accounts for nearly a fifth of global greenhouse gas emissions. As meat is such an integral part of an American diet, it's no easy feat to have everybody take responsibility and cut back. If vegetarianism isn't your thing, there are a myriad of ways to reduce your consumption, including cutting your regular meat portion in half. If the iPod-size serving is a little extreme for you to start with, a deck-of-cards-size portion should be doable for almost everybody.

BEST MEAT CHOICES

Many of us wish to continue to eat meat for enjoyment, health, or religious/cultural reasons, and there's no reason you should be forced to stop. But there are choices you can make that are healthier for you and the planet. Let's take a look at beef. Factory-farmed beef, as opposed to pasture-raised beef, is the most important meat that the Gorgeously Green Girl might want to cut back on. It is the most energy- and water-intensive food on the planet.

- Feedlot beef requires 145 times more fossil fuel to produce than potatoes.
- It takes 24 gallons of water to produce one pound of tomatoes, and 5,214 gallons of water to produce one pound of feedlot beef.
- According to the USDA, it takes sixteen pounds of grain to produce just one pound of feedlot beef.

As you can see, feedlot-beef eating consumes the world's very precious resources at an alarming rate. David Pimentel, a Cornell ecologist, says the corn we feed our feedlot cattle accounts for a staggering amount of fossil fuel energy. Growing the corn to feed livestock in this country takes vast quantities of chemical fertilizer, which requires vast quantities of oil. Because of this dependence, a typical steer will in effect consume 284 gallons of oil in his lifetime. However, not all beef is created equal. Remember, the above statistics concern themselves with *factory-farmed* or *feedlot*, not pasture-raised beef. Let rain forest burgers become a thing of the past, and if you still dream of a filet mignon, choose it wisely and save it for that extra-special occasion.

GRASS-FED BEEF

Grass-fed beef is infinitely kinder on you, the animal, and the environment. Up until the 1960s, virtually all beef was grass-fed—meaning that the cows wandered around chewing grass and thereby keeping themselves and the land healthy. After the sixties, intensive factory farming came into play, and the animals became sicker and sadder. After spending a short amount of time grazing, small calves are shoved into cramped pens and pumped with drugs to help them cope with the diseases that are caused by factory-farm conditions. Not only do you not know what you are eating when you chomp into a conventional burger or steak (you have no idea what the animal was fed), but you *can* guarantee that you are getting a hefty dose of hormones and antibiotics. Grass-fed beef is entirely different since the animals graze for their entire lives on what they were designed to eat and thus have little need for drugs to treat disease.

Grass-fed beef is much lower in fat and higher in important nutrients. It is better for the environment than factory-farmed beef because:

- There is less fuel and energy use because the animals are not raised on an energy-intensive factory farm.
- Water quality is not compromised because no chemicals are being dumped into the water supplies.

PASTURE-RAISED VERSUS FEEDLOT BEEF

Most of the meat that we see in our grocery stores is feedlot meat, meaning it has been produced in Concentrated Animal Feeding Operation (CAFO) factories, where the animals are packed together in huge numbers and fed grain instead of the grass they were designed to eat.

~ CAFOs pollute the environment with the animals' waste, whereas the waste from pasture-raised animals acts as a natural ground fertilizer.

~ CAFO animals are given growth hormones and antibiotics, whereas pasture-raised animals don't need them.

~ CAFO animal meat contains a lot of fat, owing to the grain they are fed, whereas pasture-raised animal meat is lower in fat and higher in omega-3 fatty acids, which are essential for human health.

~ CAFO animals require huge amounts of fossil fuels to rear, whereas pasture-raised animals do not.

~ A CAFO produces meat that is inferior to pasture-raised meat in quality, texture, and taste.

- Soil erosion is decreased because grass, which protects against erosion, is grown for grazing.
- The fish kill is reduced because no harmful chemicals are running into streams and lakes.
- Wildlife habitats and biodiversity are restored because of the lack of chemical pesticides.
- There's a huge reduction of antibiotics in water supplies because grass-fed animals are not injected with any drugs whatsoever.

DEMYSTIFYING MEAT LABELS

The labeling of meats can be very confusing. Should you look for "organic," "grass-fed," or just plain "natural"? It's really important that you understand your labels, as some of them have been carefully designed to confuse you.

If you want to buy meat that you can be absolutely certain has not been treated with growth hormones and/or antibiotics, your best bet is to look for meat that has a USDA "organic" label. The trouble with many of the other "no hormones/antibiotics" labels is that there is no third-party verification. This means that is it extremely unlikely that anyone will check to see if these animals aren't really being pumped full of the very things we want to avoid. We just have to take their word for it, and I'm not sure I'm willing to pay extra unless I can be sure I'm really getting what I pay for.

WHAT DO YOU WANT?

Before you go shopping, determine what you want or don't want in your meat. We all have different concerns, and with a plethora of marketing claims now flying around, we need to be clear about our needs. Do you worry about the way the animals you eat were treated? Would you rather avoid eating flesh that has been routinely injected with growth hormones? Perhaps you just want to be sure that your meat is fresh and you don't really care about the rest.

Animal welfare aside, what do we need to worry about the most? I would rather have my meat without artificial hormones. According to the European Union's Scientific Committee on Veterinary Measures Relating to Public Health, the use of growth hormones in beef production can cause a potential risk to human health.

These hormones can disrupt the *human* hormone balance, causing developmental problems, as they interfere with the reproductive system, leading to the development of breast, prostate, or colon cancer. Suffice it to say, I'll take my meat without the "growth enhancers" if possible.

What about the antibiotics? Will they end up on my plate, too? Seventy percent of antibiotics used in the United States are fed to healthy animals, as they promote growth and are a precaution against disease. The problem is that with the overuse of antibiotics, certain strains of *Salmonella, E. coli*, and other bacteria are becoming antibiotic resistant. Although it's unclear how much of the antibiotic remains in the meat on our plate, I vote with my dollars to support an industry that avoids this risky practice.

My final concern is about what the animal may have been fed. Unless you see the USDA organic label, it's likely that the meat you eat will have been fed by-products of other animals. The remains of these animals (what's not packed on a polystyrene tray and sold as meat) have to be disposed of somehow. It's typically rendered down and used as animal feed. Poultry parts are put into cattle feed and vice versa. This practice has been banned in Europe due to "mad cow" concerns, and hopefully the United States will follow.

> QUICK GUIDE
>
> **"Organic"** is the most reliable label for beef and poultry. It means the producer has had to meet a number of strict criteria, including 100-percent organic feed and no growth hormones or antibiotics, no animal by-products in the feed, and access to the outdoors.
>
> **"Certified Humane"** is the label you need to look for if you are concerned about how the animals were treated. Producers must adhere to strict animal welfare guidelines.
>
> **"Natural"** has no value as a label when it comes to meat and poultry. The animal could have eaten anything, have been fed large quantities of hormones and antibiotics, and have been badly treated.

As purchasing meat is expensive, always make a mental list of what's important to you and be sure to scrutinize the labels from now on.

DELVING DEEPER GUIDE

"No hormones added" or **"No hormones administered"**: These are labels that can be used only for beef. They are supposed to mean that no hormones have been used over the animal's lifetime. This label is only somewhat meaningful, as there is no organization behind this claim, other than the company producing or marketing the beef. Eighty percent of all U.S. feedlot cattle are injected with hormones. This label is meaningless for poultry and hogs because they are federally prohibited from being injected with hormones in the first place.

"Raised without antibiotics": This label supposedly means that throughout its lifetime, the meat or poultry has not been given any antibiotics. This label is again only somewhat meaningful because there is no third-party certifier responsible for the claim.

"Kosher": Only meat and poultry products prepared under rabbinical supervision can use this claim. This includes no environmental, health, or welfare standards (including antibiotic and hormone use).

"Humane": There is no legal or regulated definition of this claim, so different companies may use the claim to have different meanings.

"Certified humane raised and handled": This is a relatively new certification process whereby the participating companies have to adhere to a number of strict humane practices. Visit their excellent Web site for more information and to find participating companies: www.certified humane.org.

"Certified Organic": Only food producers who adhere to the USDA standards for the organic label and are certified may use this term. Organic livestock is not given antibiotics or growth hormones and is fed only organically produced feed and must have access to pasture. Organic meat cannot be irradiated.

"Grass-fed": The USDA has issued a proposed standard that will require the label "grass-fed" to mean "100 percent grass-fed," but this label is tricky for a number of reasons. There is no third-party verification, and apparently some producers use this popular label despite the fact that the animals have been fed grain for a large proportion of their lives. Further, the animals may have been injected with hormones and antibiotics. Finally, don't assume that the "grass-fed" label means Rosie the cow was treated lovingly her whole life long—she may have been fed grass while being confined in a barn with dozens of her unhappy friends.

"Free Range": The USDA allows producers to put this label on products made from poultry that have been allowed outside access. This could simply mean a small open door or window in an overly crowded barn. There is no third-party verification, so you just have to trust that the door was left open!

"Fresh" means very little as far as meat is concerned. It's simply a legal meaning that the food in question has not been frozen (below 26 degrees F).

"No Additives" just means that one of the 2,800 USDA-listed chemical substances has not been used to give the meat a "technical effect." This includes coloring, flavoring, and preservatives.

The answer is to cut down on your meat, and when you do buy it, try to give yourself and your family the best, which should bear the certified organic label. You will be doing your body and the planet a massive favor by avoiding feedlot beef completely. Avoiding cruelty, hormones, and environmental devastation is paramount when choosing beef.

Tip: Since grass-fed beef has a slightly different taste, try introducing it slowly into your diet. A good starting point would be to add it to a Bolognese sauce, a stew, or a chili.

As organic beef is more expensive, I recommend saving it for a treat. If you are eating it twice a month instead of every day, your budget should allow for eating meat that is kinder to your body and the environment.

WHERE CAN I FIND IT?

Armed with all the above labeling information, you can now scout out the availability of quality meat in your area. I recommend asking a lot of questions. If your local health food store has a meat section, find out the name of the meat supplier and look up its Web site. You could always pick up the phone and call. The best thing you can do is to actually get to know a meat supplier. There are many wonderful meat producers who adhere to all of the "organic" criteria and yet, for a number of reasons, don't have the USDA certification. If they are transparent enough to allow you to visit their farm or sufficiently answer your questions, you may be satisfied.

A fantastic Web site with all kinds of information about grass-fed meat is www.eatwild.com. You can click on their map to find a producer near you.

I also recommend visiting www.localharvest.org. Click on "farm" and enter your choice of meat (beef, poultry, or pork). Finally, enter your zip code, and all your nearest farms will be listed.

To purchase great beef, try:
www.nimanranch.com

www.certified-organic-beef.com
www.grasslandbeef.com

For money-saving coupons, visit www.gorgeouslygreen.com/coupons.

BISON AND BUFFALO

You can be pretty sure that if you buy bison or buffalo, these animals will have been grass-fed. They are basically wild animals that graze out on huge open pastures. The meat is absolutely delicious—very similar to beef, but a little sweeter. It is cost-effective because the meat is so dense that you need only half the amount you would normally eat of, say, a steak. It is very low in fat. It is a heritage animal, meaning that when we first came to America, these animals were roaming literally *everywhere*. Go to this excellent Web site to read more about one particularly fantastic producer: www.lindnerbison.com.

CHICKEN AND TURKEY

Americans eat double the amount of chicken that we used to eat twenty years ago. It's often touted as a great diet food, for it's a lean and relatively healthy form of protein. What is chicken's eco-impact? Most chicken in the United States is raised in huge concentrated feeding operations. Their feed is laced with artificial hormones, antibiotics, animal by-products, fish, and even arsenic. The birds are debeaked and often diseased from their cramped living quarters, and obviously suffer horribly. Unless the chicken you buy is labeled "Certified Organic," it's likely to have come from one of these unpleasant establishments. If you are buying case-ready chicken breasts, they have probably been pumped full of saline to appear juicier than they are (that's why they shrink so much during cooking). Don't forget that the polystyrene and plastic wrap packaging could leak harmful chemicals into the flesh, and it is not recyclable. Suffice it to say, it's a good idea for your health and the planet that you buy certified organic chicken or at least chicken that is hormone- and antibiotic-free.

It's pretty much the same deal with turkey, that wondrous bird that used to be reserved for a Thanksgiving treat. The turkey that our great-grandparents ate was very different from the ubiquitous dry white bird we eat today. There were hundreds of breeds, and each region used to favor its own particular one. Today, these breeds are known as "heritage" turkeys and they are making a comeback, thanks to organizations like www.heritageturkeyfoundation.org. You can order a heritage turkey from www.heritagefoodsusa.com and have it shipped overnight to you. Heritage turkeys actually taste of turkey and are much more succulent and delicious. They are expensive, but for a once-a-year treat, it's worth it.

Regular turkey has become a daily deli staple for many, and particularly for those on diets, so try to avoid it unless it satisfies your Gorgeously Green criteria.

Petaluma Poultry is a great resource for finding certified organic chicken and other meats. They were the first company to get organic certification, for their "Rosie" chicken. They have a store locator at www.petalumapoultry.com.

LAMB AND PORK

Americans don't eat as much pork as they did two decades ago, except in the form of bacon. Bacon has become a condiment, added to everything from salads to omelets. The problem is that most bacon, unless otherwise stated on the packet, contains nitrates (preservatives), which have been linked to cancer. Nitrates are found in many cured meats, including hams, salamis, and especially hot dogs.

Look for nitrate-free organic bacon, hot dogs, and cold cuts.

Lamb is a good meat choice because it is less intensively farmed in the United States. Much of our lamb comes from New Zealand, which has strict rules about how the animals are raised. New Zealand legislation does not permit the use of growth hormones. However, it does have to travel a long way, so I prefer to find reliable organic U.S.-reared lamb. See www.nimanranch.com.

Since eating meat isn't the most eco-friendly activity on earth, I have included two or three meat-free days in the Light and Bright Green plans. The Deep Green eating plan is 100-percent vegetarian. Remember, the Gorgeously Green Diet is not about being extreme; it is rather about making small changes that will add up to your feeling better all the way around. Small incremental steps always work, and cutting your meat eating by half is easier than cutting your driving time by half.

BEST DAIRY CHOICES

MILK

What about dairy? How do my latte and grilled cheese sandwich affect my eco-impact, never mind my potentially bulging thighs? The way that conventional milk is produced is no different from the horrors found in feedlot beef farms. The conditions in conventional dairy farms can be apalling. Many people won't eat dairy products because they are disgusted at the way many dairy animals are treated. Large corporate-owned factories pack the cows into massive warehouses and treat them simply as milk machines. It's common for them to be forced to produce 100 pounds of milk a day—ten times more than they would produce naturally. They are artificially inseminated and, owing to growth hormones and unnatural milking schedules, their udders get painful and so swollen that they drag on the ground. This increases the chance of infection and overuse of antibiotics. If this kind of abuse is a particular concern of yours, go to www.americanhumane.org and find out if there is a certified humane dairy producer near you. To get this certification, producers have to treat their animals *really* well.

> **WHAT IS rBGH?**
>
> It stands for recombinant bovine growth hormone. Cows in large factory farms are injected with it to increase their milk production by up to 40 percent. All dairy milk in America is genetically modified in this way, except that labeled "no rBGH" or "rBGH-free." The Cancer Prevention Coalition (www.preventcancer.com), an organization founded by Samuel Epstein, MD, an expert on the causes and prevention of cancer, believes that bovine growth hormone in milk increases the risk of cancer in humans. It is currently banned in Europe.

The other concern that many people have with dairy is that it will pack on the pounds. However, fat does not equal "fat" if it's the right kind of fat. There have been numerous peer-reviewed scientific studies proving that eating the right kinds of fat can help you lose weight. *Raw* milk, butter, and cream are on my "healthy" fats list. Almost all the milk you buy in a store, even organic milk, is pasteurized. Pasteurization kills friendly bacteria and greatly diminishes the nutritional content of the milk. It destroys phosphatase, which is essential for the absorption of calcium, and kills lipase (an enzyme unique to milk and needed to complete digestion of the fat in the milk). This is why I prefer raw milk and am lucky enough to be able to buy it in the state of California. It is illegal to sell raw milk in eighteen U.S. states, and people are understandably cautious about its safety. If you want to read more about the benefits of raw milk, visit www.westonprice.org, and if you want to find a reliable and safe source in your state, visit www.realmilk.com.

If you feel more comfortable with pasteurized milk, make absolutely sure that it's labeled organic or "rBGH-free."

The practice of injecting animals with growth hormones is also bad for the environment because when these poor cows are forced to unnaturally increase milk production, they need to eat a lot more food. This means that more farmland is planted with genetically modified crops that are sprayed with pesticides and herbicides, which in turn pollute our waterways.

Suffice it to say, always look for hormone-free milk. The good news is that you should be able to find it in most large grocery chains.

Since my family consumes a little milk every day, I buy organic milk, which means that it is not only hormone-free but also that the cow has had access to the outdoors and has been fed an organic diet.

In the Coffee Shop

When you go to the coffee shop, ask what kind of milk they use because you don't want to be getting a "grande" load of hormones in your double skinny latte. Many of the large coffee-shop chains have committed to using hormone-free milk, but it's taking them a while to implement this change, so be sure to ask. Even better, brew your own organic coffee at home because:

- It could save you up to $1,200 a year.
- You won't be using one of the 28 billion paper cups that are trashed every year in the United States.
- You can brew premium-grade organic coffee and use organic milk for a tenth of the price of a lower-quality coffee-shop drink.

What's the difference in labeling between organic and rBGH-free milk?

The USDA has established rules so you can understand the difference.

USDA regulations for **organic** milk prohibit the use of artificial growth hormones and antibiotics, while mandating that cows are given access to pasture and are fed organic grains.

Dairies that produce and market hormone-free milk have essentially agreed to abide by just one of the principles of organic milk production.

While "organic" dairy farmers have to be inspected by independent third parties who verify a farmer's compliance, "hormone-free" dairy farms are not inspected. In most cases, those farmers sign a legally binding affidavit instead.

Best Milk Choices

The best choice is **whole organic raw milk** because you'll be getting all the nutrients you need plus the enzymes needed to digest the fat. You may be freaking out, for it's likely that any diet you have ever tried has prescribed nonfat milk. It's the common assumption that full-cream milk and dairy products are the predominant cause of hefty thighs and heart disease. Recent scientific research has shown, however, that the correlation between saturated fats and heart disease may be misleading.

The fats that we really need to avoid are fats that have been hydrogenated or partially hydrogenated. These are called trans fats and are believed to lower our good cholesterol and increase our triglycerides, which can lead to heart disease. Although some restaurant chains have now banned trans fats, you should still be wary. Labels can say "0 grams of trans fat" even if partially hydrogenated fats are in the ingredient list. If the serving contains less than 0.5 grams of trans fats, manufacturers can use this label. However, the problem is that if anyone eats more than a single serving (which most people do), these fractional amounts of trans fats can add up. The unadulterated fats found in beautiful raw and nonhomogenized dairy products will do you no such harm.

Many health food stores now carry raw milk from reputable dairies, in glass bottles. It takes a little getting used to, since it is much creamier than regular milk and has a shorter shelf life. A useful tip is to spoon off the thick cream and put it aside for cooking or your coffee.

Homogenized milk has been heat-blasted to disperse the fat throughout the milk instead of letting it rise to the top. Unfortunately, this process is highly controversial, for it is believed by many to be a cause of heart disease. If you can't get raw milk, I recommend trying to find **organic nonhomogenized milk** in glass bottles. You can assume that most milk in grocery stores is homogenized, unless otherwise stated. You may have to check out your local health food store to find the non–heat-blasted version. Either it will come in a glass bottle so that you can see that the cream has risen to the top (a sign that it has not been homogenized), or it will be clearly labeled as "nonhomogenized." It is sometimes labeled as "cream on top" milk. Straus Family Farms carries milk that has been pasteurized at 170 degrees F for only nineteen seconds, as opposed to regular organic milk, which is heated to 280 degrees F for two to four seconds. This means that the Straus milk retains many more nutrients and enzymes. Visit www.strausfamilycreamery.com to see if your local store carries this brand.

Organic Valley (www.organicvalleycoop.com) carries nonhomogenized milk. You'll find not only a store locator on their Web site but also money-off coupons.

Many grocery store chains, including Trader Joe's, have their own brands of organic milk at a pretty reasonable price. Always look for specials.

Goat milk is a great choice if you can deal with the "goat" taste. It is almost always organic and the goats are never treated with growth hormones. It's one of the easiest milks for humans to digest—easier than cow's milk. If you are lactose intolerant, you'll be fine with this choice. Many good grocery chains carry Meyenberg Goat Milk Products (www.meyenberg.com), and if you do like goat milk, treat yourself to some incredible LãLoo's goat milk ice cream (www.goatmilkicecream.com).

If you like **half & half** in your coffee, make sure that it's organic, too. **Whole milk** is far superior to reduced-fat or nonfat milk since it contains the enzymes you need for digestion. There is obviously a little more fat in it, but, in small quantities, this healthy fat will not harm you.

Nondairy milk/creamer: As I suggest using milk in moderation, a healthy alternative for you and the planet would be **organic rice, almond, or hemp milk**. I like Rice Dream and Wild Harvest (www.wildharvestorganic.com), which can be found at many large grocery stores. Pacific Natural Foods (www.pacificfoods.com) carries a great selection of nut beverages. Visit their Web site for a store locator. Visit www.manitobaharvest.com for hemp milk.

In a pinch, www.diamondorganics.com will overnight any organic dairy product to you, and they carry all of the brands that I recommend.

Finally, the most eco-friendly option is to always buy your milk in glass bottles that are returnable. The waxed milk cartons are generally not recyclable, so if you do get them, go to www.earth911.com to see if your municipality accepts them in your curbside recycling bin.

BEST CHEESE AND YOGURT CHOICES

Look for the same labeling as discussed for milk. Yogurt, sour cream, kefir, cheese, cottage cheese, and heavy cream will have the same labeling. Keep in mind that the same companies that eschew hormones in their milk may still use them to produce their cheese products. So scrutinize those labels.

I'm in love with **kefir**—it tastes very similar to yogurt and comes in a variety of delicious flavors. It is fermented milk with a plethora of health benefits, including antibiotic and antifungal properties, and promotes healthy gut flora. Many doctors believe that good health begins in the gut. Your colon contains billions of microbes, some good and some bad. A healthy gut depends on a balance of good and bad, and too many "bad" microbes can create toxins and cause us to get sick. Probiotics lower the pH of the colon, which helps the good microbes and hinders the bad. This can help boost your immune system. The correct balance of healthy bacteria can also help us to absorb our food. No wonder the word *kefir* was derived from the Turkish word *keif,* which means "good feeling." I suggest trying some and, if you like it, eat a little a day, either in place of yogurt or in a smoothie. I recommend Lifeway Kefir, as they have several different fruit blends and a nondairy kefir, too. On their Web site, www.lifeway.net, there's a store locator. You'll also find kefir in the yogurt section of many grocery stores.

Buying **yogurt** can be really confusing because of all the silly marketing claims that are prevalent on virtually every container. We are now being told that certain yogurts can provide our daily fiber requirements, boost our immune system, and remove cholesterol. I suggest going for plain yogurt with only two ingredients: live cultures and milk. A long list of ingredients probably includes emulsifiers, stabilizers, sugar, and so on. I prefer whole-milk yogurts, for I eat only a little and much prefer the taste and texture. However, there are some fantastic low-fat Greek yogurts that are just as creamy as full-fat yogurt. Yogurt is often digestible for even those of you with lactose intolerance. I love using it as a substitute for mayonnaise and as a delicious addition to many recipes.

The best option to reduce your eco-impact is to make your own yogurt, which is very easy and will save you a considerable amount of money as well as packaging. If you do buy store-bought yogurt, *always* pick the largest container you can find and remember to recycle the pot. I strongly advise you not to buy the tubes of yogurt for your kids because they always contain sugar, and the individual packaging is not eco-friendly. I add fresh fruit to my homemade yogurt and put it in a little thermos flask for my daughter's school lunch box.

I recommend both Stonyfield and Horizon yogurts, which are available at most large grocery stores.

www.stonyfield.com
www.horizon.com

I also love Nancy's organic yogurt (www.nancysyogurt.com).

Greek yogurt is an excellent choice because it is so thick and creamy. I use Greek yogurt for cooking and adding to all kinds of dishes, from baked yams to soups.

I love Oikos Organic Greek Yogurt (www.oikosyogurt.com) and Fage (www.fageusa.com).

I include a lot of goat cheese in the eating plan because it is easier to digest than other cheese. However, if you don't like the taste, pick out a cheese that you love and, if possible, buy it raw. Cheese made of sheep's milk is extremely nutritious; it has a high proportion of short- and medium-chain fatty acids, which don't affect cholesterol levels and make the milk very easy to digest. It's more expensive than cow's milk because the dairy sheep industry is in its infancy in the United States. If you're going to eat cheese, eat it as the French do (remember, French women don't get fat!), without bread and in small, one-ounce (two-dice) portions. Most grocery stores now boast a decent collection of organic cheeses and some wonderful goat cheese options.

Be really careful when buying nondairy or soy cheese, for it often contains sugar, high-fructose corn syrup, and other questionable additives to make it taste even half decent.

I use a little butter, but I primarily use **ghee**, which is just like clarified butter and is simply delicious. It is the rich, golden butterfat that is left when the milk solids are removed. You can buy it in jars at health food stores, but it's honestly so easy to make that you should save your money (see page 172). It's used in Indian and French cuisine and is wonderful for frying because it doesn't burn. It has a bucketload of health benefits and is lactose-free.

BEST EGG CHOICES

You can buy eggs from "humane" producers, and unless you are vegan, you shouldn't be afraid of this wonderfood, which contains *every* nutrient the body needs with the exception of vitamin C. The yolk contains special fatty acids that are necessary for nerve function, and the whites are the highest-quality protein you can find.

WHAT ABOUT DHA- OR OMEGA-3-ENRICHED EGGS?

A great option for getting some healthy omega-3 fatty acids into your diet is to buy eggs that are enriched with them. Remember, omega-3 fatty acids are the essential fatty acids that we must get from our diet. As the typical American diet is lacking in these vital nutrients, it will behoove you to choose foods that you know contain them. Current research findings suggest that omega-3 fatty acids play a role in reducing the risk of heart disease. Omega-3-enriched eggs are produced by altering the diet of laying hens. The hens are fed a special diet, which contains 10–20 percent ground flaxseed. Flaxseed is higher in omega-3 fatty acids and lower in saturated fatty acids than any other grain.

ORGANIC EGGS

Buying eggs can be very confusing because of the plethora of options. I pay extra and get certified organic eggs because I believe that the quality of the yolk is directly affected by what the bird ate. I also couldn't bear to think that my sunny-side up came from a brutally treated hen!

"Certified Organic": The birds are uncaged and fed an organic vegetarian diet.

"Certified humane": The birds are uncaged and must be able to engage in natural behavior. This label doesn't specify diet.

"Cage-free": The birds are uncaged, but they are not guaranteed outside access, and this label doesn't specify diet.

"Vegetarian-fed": The birds have a more "natural" diet, but this label says nothing about their living conditions, so you are likely getting eggs from a battery hen.

LOCALLY PRODUCED EGGS

Your best and least expensive bet is to try to find locally produced eggs. Many farmers sell their eggs at farmer's markets and you can check out your nearest community supported agriculture (CSA). I suggest visiting the great Web site www.localharvest.org to see if any farms in your area provide this service, where for a small annual fee you can buy a "share" of the farm, so that meat, dairy, and/or produce will be available to you year-round. Simply enter your zip code and what you are looking to buy.

I recommend the following brands, which you will find in most large grocery chains:

Horizon (www.horizon.com)
Organic Valley (www.organicvalley.coop)
Wild Harvest Organic (www.wildharvestorganic.com)
Whole Foods 365 store brand

If my yard were even a few square feet larger, I'd keep a few chickens—but the idea of that, coupled with my rather excellent plan of converting our front yard into an "edible" yard, was somewhat poorly received by my husband, who wondered how on earth I would be able to work with chickens when I have a pathological fear of pecking beaks. I countered with the fact that I am also terrified of rats and that I've had to face that fear with the compost bin, which I have to whack with a long pole before I get anywhere near it, to ensure that Rosemary, our new backyard rat, isn't lurking.

BEST OIL CHOICES

The most important thing to consider is *what* you are using the oil for. You should use different oil for cooking and frying than you do for dressings and sauces. This is because of the smoke-point issue. Every unrefined vegetable oil has a natural "smoke point," which is the temperature to which it can be heated before it starts decomposing or burning. Many vegetable oils are refined to increase their smoke point and make them suitable for cooking at high temperatures. Refined oils have been:

- Treated with chemical solvents
- Heated to an extremely high temperature, causing the formation of trans-fatty acids, which have been linked to heart disease and cancer.

This leaves us with a conundrum—what on earth should we fry our onions in? The answer is to "steam-fry" as much as possible. I use chicken or vegetable broth instead of oil to begin with (until the onions are soft), and then I add a little olive oil.

We are encouraged by most of the country's top chefs to sling a bit of EVOO (extra-virgin olive oil) into a skillet to fry just about everything. However, I disagree. Most of my friends in Italy never fry with extra virgin olive oil because it has a relatively low smoke point and is far too expensive to be wasted on frying. Instead they use either pure olive oil (see below) or canola oil and then finish off the dish with the EVOO.

Here are the different kinds of olive oil you can buy:

- Extra-virgin: Considered the best, this oil comes from the first pressing of the olives and is usually cold-pressed.
- Virgin: This oil comes from the second pressing.
- Pure: This undergoes some processing, such as filtering and refining.
- Extra light: This oil undergoes considerable processing and retains only a very mild olive flavor.

An even bigger problem is that most extra-virgin olive oil sold in large grocery chain stores is not what they would have you believe it to be. Except in California, the labeling laws allow for adulterated olive oils to be called "extra-virgin." Many of the large Italian manufacturers dilute their olive oil with cheap hazelnut oil from Turkey. They estimate they can add up to 20 percent of a nut oil without the consumer being able to detect it. It now makes sense why so many stores carry enormous liter bottles of ostensibly extra-virgin olive oil for a low price. So, unless you live in California, where manufacturers are forced to label honestly, you may have to do some research. High-quality EVOO contains flavonoids, polyphenols, and squalene—all of which help protect against cancer. This is why proper olive oil is one of the healthiest oils you can eat. Use it generously in dressings and homemade mayonnaise, or to drizzle over veggies. Here are a few of my trusted resources:

> ### STEAM-FRYING
>
> Frying onions, garlic, or a variety of vegetables forms the base for many of the recipes included in the Gorgeously Green Diet.
>
> If the recipe tells you to heat 2 tablespoons of olive oil, you can substitute with 4 tablespoons of vegetable or chicken broth. This is a good tip for weight loss as well as your health.

- www.cooc.com: The California Olive Oil Council is a nonprofit that offers an independent seal-of-approval certification to various producers, making sure you get the real thing.
- www.oliveoilsource.com: This excellent Web site lists all the main U.S. olive oil manufacturers and states whether or not they are certified.
- www.figueroafarms.com: This is a family-run business that produces the most exquisite, award-winning extra-virgin olive oil. These oils are an absolute treat and make a wonderful hostess gift.
- www.wildernessfamilynaturals.com: This company carries a beautiful raw, certified organic olive oil.
- www.edenfoods.com: This is one of my favorite companies for just about everything and they carry a wonderful extra-virgin olive oil from Spain. Check the store locator on their site.

Tip: Sunlight can oxidize your olive oil and turn it rancid quickly. Always make sure your olive oil comes in a dark glass bottle to protect it from light, and keep it in a cool, dark cupboard.

Best Oils for Frying

1. Pure olive oil (not EVOO). Smoke point: 438 degrees F
2. Grape seed oil. Smoke point: 420 degrees F
3. Virgin coconut oil. Smoke point: 350 degrees F
4. Expeller-pressed canola oil. Smoke point: 400 degrees F

An excellent source for all these oils is www.spectrumorganics.com.

BEST COFFEE AND TEA CHOICES

If you love coffee, you'll be thrilled to realize that you can still have it on this plan, but it's best to limit yourself to *one or two* cups a day, because too much caffeine can deplete your body of calcium and make you jittery and irritable. Make sure you buy **organic and fair-trade** coffee; it is kinder to the environment and the people who produce it. Coffee and tea contain many antioxidants, so they can be good for you in moderation.

I love these brands:

- Good Earth Coffee (www.goodearthcoffee.com) is great since it's organic, widely available in many large grocery chains, and reasonably priced.
- Equal Exchange (www.equalexchange.coop) is organic and fair-trade coffee, which is also available nationally.

Look for store-brand organic coffee, which is often on sale.

If you go to the coffee shop, try to order organic coffee and remember that they probably won't be using organic milk or creamer. Avoid the ice-blended drinks and smoothies; they are made with mixes that are packed with sugar and additives. Finally, take a reusable cup with you and remember that too many visits can get pretty costly, and this eating plan is about wise budgeting. Brewing a cup of beautiful organic coffee at home will cost you less than a quarter, whereas daily trips to the café could add up to the price of a nice designer outfit every month.

It's more eco-friendly to use a coffee machine that doesn't require paper filters. If you do use them, however, make sure you buy the unbleached ones, because the manufacturing process is much kinder to the planet. Every industrial process that involves chlorine bleach spews out toxic emissions called dioxins, which have been linked to cancer.

Never drink coffee or tea from polystyrene cups. They cannot be recycled. If you visit a shop or a restaurant that still uses them, I dare you to muster up the courage to have a word with the manager—I often do this, but I try to be charming about it with something like, "I just love this restaurant and since I am attempting to go green, would you be open to investigating an alterative to using polystyrene cups?" I have had some wonderful results with this approach, especially one manager who said he would be thrilled if I would e-mail him some more eco-friendly options. That afternoon, he had the information in hand, and about a month later, he had made the switch. I wanted to hug him. If you want to pass on these resources to your local coffee shop or restaurant, here they are:

www.letsgogreen.biz
www.greenlinepaper.com

Green tea has many health benefits. It contains a class of polyphenols (antioxidants) called catechins, which studies have shown can inhibit disease-promoting inflammatory compounds and boost your immune system. Research has also shown that it can increase your metabolism, strengthen your bones, and prevent tooth decay—so I've become a passionate Gorgeously Green tea drinker. I highly recommend the Strand Tea Company (www.strandtea.com). This company carries an incredible selection of every kind of tea imaginable. They are extremely eco-conscious with a strong commitment to social responsibility. If you are new to green tea, consider purchasing a tea sampler from them and keep in mind that the best-quality tea is always loose tea, as opposed to tea bags. Strand Tea also carries some great accessories for loose tea, including the "Tea Tiger," a fantastic thermal travel mug with a built-in filter.

You can also find a great selection of organic green teas in most large grocery chains. I like:

Tazo Tea (www.tazotea.com)
Numi Tea (www.numitea.com)
Celestial Seasoning's Organic Green Tea (www.celestialseasonings.com)
Yogi Tea (www.yogitea.com)

You can buy teas in bulk from a huge selection at www.mountainroseherbs.com.

I also love matcha Green Tea. The entire leaf is ground into a bright, green powder, which you can make into a creamy latte (www.domatcha.com).

PROTEIN BARS AND DRINKS

I'm not a huge fan of protein bars, because I think it's better to meet your protein needs with "real" foods. However, for many vegans, vegetarians, and those of us who are on the road, we sometimes need to find a convenient, effective, and, hopefully, delicious way to get our daily protein requirements met.

Be really careful when buying protein bars and powders. They can contain a host of additives that are horrible. I recommend eating **soy protein isolate** very sparingly (see box). If you do buy soy isolate powder, make absolutely sure that you see the USDA organic label, because many conventional powders contain hexane, a petroleum solvent that has adverse effects on you and your environment.

I prefer whey protein powder to soy. It's more easily digested, even for those who have an intolerance to regular dairy products. It doesn't contain casein, which is the substance in many dairy products that most people find hard to digest. Always check that this powder is organic and doesn't contain any additives.

> ### SOY PROTEIN ISOLATE (SPI)
>
> SPI is a highly processed food. The soybeans are acid-washed in aluminum tanks, which leach high levels of aluminum (a neurotoxin) into the final product. Nitrites, potent carcinogens, are formed during the spray-drying phase that turns the curds into high-protein powder. A toxic amino acid called lysinoalanine is formed during the subsequent alkaline processing.
>
> Finally, numerous artificial flavorings (including MSG) are often added to the final product. What winds up in the large plastic tubs in your health food store may not be as good for your body and the environment as you thought.

By far the best protein powder is **hemp**—it is always organic, contains all the amino acids you need, and is extremely high in protein. It is also easily digested. You can find a large selection of hemp bars and powders at www.nutiva.com.

The following are my favorite protein bars and will work really well for the office girl:

1. **Whey Proteins Green Plus** taste great. They are packed with superfoods, which are fantastically healthy, and contain sixteen grams of protein. They are relatively high in calories, so cut the bar in half if you aren't moving around too much that day (www.greensplus.com).
2. **Vega Whole Food Raw Energy Bar** tastes scrumptious and will give you ten grams of wonderful hemp protein (www.veganessentials.com).

3. **Jay Robb** bars are all utterly delicious and contain fourteen grams of protein—made with whey protein and all good stuff (www.jayrobb.com).
4. **Think Organic** and **Think Green** carry delicious fruity bars. Great for a little afternoon pick-me-up (www.thinkproducts.com).

I have included a whey or hemp protein powder in all of the plans. Here are the brands I recommend:

www.jayrobb.com
www.energyfirst.com
www.livingharvest.com
www.manitobaharvest.com

I have also included **green superfoods** to add to your smoothies. Green super-foods are phytonutrient-rich green plants, algae, and cereal grasses. They are an excellent source of vitamins, minerals, amino acids, enzymes, and plant sterols. I don't like the taste, so I disguise it by mixing them into yummy smoothies. You can also take them in capsule form. Here are my favorites:

www.amazinggrass.com
www.synergy-co.com

The most eco-friendly thing you can do is to make your own energy/protein bars at home (see the recipes section). It will save money and landfill packaging!

SWEETENERS

Whichever way you want to skin the cat, sugar is sugar, regardless of the form it comes in. The only difference between the white, refined stuff and the sweeteners listed below is that the regular sugar doesn't contain one single nutrient—so you are eating an empty, blood-sugar-spiking, turn-straight-to-fat-on-the-thighs substance!

I recommend sticking to the most natural sweeteners you can find. My all-time favorite is **stevia**, which is made from the stevia plant and has no carbs whatsoever, plus a rating of zero on the glycemic index. The glycemic index (GI) measures the effects of carbohydrates on blood glucose levels. The lower a rating, the healthier a food is considered to be. Stevia also contains fiber, which helps with weight loss. Use only a tiny amount, for it's a gazillion times sweeter than sugar.

Organic Zero (www.wholesomesweeteners.com) is produced from organic cane sugar juice, naturally fermented and crystallized to create organic erythritol, a sugar alcohol that occurs naturally in fruits and veggies and even in our bodies! It looks very similar to table sugar but is 70 percent as sweet. I like that it has a glycemic index of zero and virtually no calories.

Honey has more calories than refined sugar, but it has more nutrients and contains small amounts of trace minerals. Always buy raw organic honey, since conventionally produced honey has been found to contain high levels of pesticides. You can find a wonderful raw honey at www.tropicaltraditions.com. Raw honey also doesn't spike blood sugar in the same way that regular sugar does, and scientific research has found it to contain probiotics, which help to increase the good bacteria (bifidobacteria and lactobacilli) in your gut, leading to a healthier digestive system. Raw honey is simply honey that is not produced using the high temperatures typically used in honey extraction and production. The lower temperatures ensure that the beneficial enzymes stay intact. It's slower and more laborious to produce and so can be more expensive.

Manuka Honey is exclusively from New Zealand, where the bees feed on the native tea tree (*Malaleuca alternifolia*) bush. This extraordinary honey has been found to have medicinal properties. With a UMF (unique manuka factor) of between 16 and 18, this honey can help with all kinds of conditions, from heartburn, stomach ulcers, and sore throats to external wounds. To establish the UMF of the honey, clinical trials measure its antibacterial efficiency by comparing it with a standard antiseptic in its ability to fight bacteria. It is absolutely delicious, and I often give Lola a teaspoon in her oatmeal during the winter months. It's expensive, so you may not want to use it on your breakfast toast every day. But always keep a jar handy (www.manukahoney.com).

Brown rice syrup is one of my favorite sweeteners. I use it for baking or to pour over ice cream or pancakes. It is thick and honey-colored and has a caramel-malt taste (www.lundberg.com).

Maple syrup is obviously from the maple tree and is delectable, but do make sure that you are getting the real thing. Many regular grocery stores carry imitation maple syrup that is full of additives. I love a producer called the Coombs Family Farms, because they are involved with environmental stewardship and sustainable forestry (www.coombsfamilyfarms.com).

Unsulfured molasses is a wonderful sweetener for baking. It contains iron, potassium, magnesium, and calcium. You can buy it at most good grocery and health food stores.

Xylitol is a sugar alcohol that is absorbed more slowly than sugar, so it doesn't cause the blood-sugar spikes that regular sugar does. Xylosweet, which can be purchased at www.xlear.com or at most health food stores, can be used as a regular sweetener. You can also find it in candy, chewing gum, and dental products, as it has been found to be beneficial for teeth.

Finally, *avoid* artificial/chemical sweeteners at all costs: **Aspartame, Nutrasweet**, **Equal,** and **Splenda.** Although they have been approved for safety by the FDA, 85 percent of *all* complaints coming into the FDA are from people suffering from adverse reactions to one of these chemical sweeteners. They are in everything from breath mints to sodas to yogurts—so keep an eagle eye out for these highly controversial chemicals. If you have a sweet tooth, be really safe and use one of the sweeteners mentioned above instead. I'd rather have my yummy sweets from a recognizable plant or tree than from a laboratory. According to the Feingold Association, an organization that educates parents about the effects of food additives (www.feingold.org), doctors have reported many cases in which patients have gained significant amounts of weight after they began using synthetic sweeteners. It is theorized that the chemicals interfere with the body's ability to signal when it is satisfied. Aspartame is suspected of interfering with the production of serotonin (a neurotransmitter, which is involved in sleep, memory, mood, and other neurological processes) and the release of insulin.

BREADS/CRACKERS/PASTA/CEREALS

Refined flours and sugars are bad for your health and the environment. The industrial process used to refine these foods requires a great deal of fossil fuel and synthetic chemicals, and creates waste. White flour is what is left after whole-grain wheat has been stripped of the very nutrients and fiber that we depend on for optimal health and a strong digestive system. White flour is not a living food. It is an empty calorie that will spike your blood sugar without giving you any nutrients in return. This spike in blood sugar not only leads to the excess glucose being stored as fat but also causes your blood sugar to plummet, leaving you wanting more. Foods were initially refined to extend their shelf life, but we have paid a very high price to enable the food industry to achieve its goal of a white loaf that lasts for weeks. I bake my own whole-wheat bread, and without refrigeration, it lasts for about three days. Most baked goods that are made of white flour also contain a host of unhealthy additives. Consuming healthy fats with your grains will actually lower their glycemic index—if you spread butter on your whole-grain toast, the fat will slow down the rate at which the sugar is absorbed into your bloodstream. That's good news for a girl who likes nothing better than a slice of hot buttered toast on a cold morning.

I love sprouted-grain bread because the process of sprouting the grains makes them more digestible. The sprouting process converts the natural starches in the grains into digestible, simple vegetable sugars, so your body recognizes and digests sprouted grains as it would a vegetable. Sprouting the grains also increases their vitamin and enzyme content. Food for Life (www.food forlife.com) makes the most delicious sprouted-grain breads: I love their Ezekiel 4:9 breads. They are a little firmer than a regular bread, so they work best if you keep them in the fridge and then toast. Food for Life also carries sprouted-grain tortillas, which are wonderful for making wraps. Their Web site has a store locator; you'll find that their products are widely available.

> ### BREAD ADDITIVES TO AVOID
>
> Since the Gorgeously Green Diet is about eating fresh and minimally processed foods, it will behoove you to avoid the following additives. Many of them have been found to cause allergic reactions or to aggravate existing allergies.
>
> Potassium bromate
> Calcium propionate
>
> Also avoid partially hydrogenated oils and high-fructose corn syrup. These are the culprits that can easily lead to heart disease, obesity, and cancer.

If you are looking for **whole wheat bread** in the grocery store, don't be fooled by all the claims on the package. The label must say "whole wheat flour" and have it listed as the *first* ingredient. Most bread in grocery chains is made with refined white flour, even if they say:

- Wheat flour
- Unbleached wheat flour
- Unbleached enriched white flour

Crackers are an additive minefield, too—they generally contain way too many syrups and unhealthy oils. Crackers and chips are a very dense carbohydrate, so if you want to avoid packing on the pounds, eat them only occasionally, and when you do, pick one of the following brands, most of which are widely available in grocery stores:

Ry Krisp
Finn Crisp
Kavli flatbreads
Archer Farms organic crackers (at Target)
Kashi TLC seven-grain crackers

Check the store locator for my three all-time favorite crackers/chips:

Mary's Gone Crackers (www.marysgonecrackers.com)
Doctor Kracker (www.drkracker.com)
Lundberg Original Sea Salt Rice Chips (www.lundberg.com)

PASTA

Who doesn't adore **pasta**? I could eat a bowl almost every night, and it's easy and inexpensive. The best pastas are made from high-quality durum wheat, which is the hardest of all wheats and has a very high protein and gluten content, which makes it ideal for pasta. Cheaper brands use soft-wheat flour that falls apart or becomes gluey when cooked. Look for pasta that has a rich, yellow color as opposed to white, an indication that the better durum wheat is being used. Although Italians would be horrified, I do suggest eating whole-grain pasta if you're worried about your blood sugar spiking. I also love to experiment with pastas that mix in other grains, such as buckwheat with the durum wheat. Many of these pastas have a complex, nutty taste and work well with really simple sauces. The following companies have a great selection of organic pastas:

Eden Foods (www.edenfoods.com)
DeBoles Pasta (www.deboles.com)

You can also find some excellent store-brand organic pastas in most large grocery chains.

Quinoa (KEEN-wah) is one of my all-time favorite grains. It's extremely high in protein and has a lovely nutty taste. It actually has the best amino-acid profile of any grain. Quinoa is known as the "mother grain" in South America and has been used for more than five thousand years as a great source of protein. I have included the grains and the pasta in your eating plans. You can buy the organic grains at www .whitemountainfarm.com or you can find the pasta at:

Andean Dream (www.andeandream.com). This is my favorite quinoa pasta. It is made only from organic royal quinoa and rice flour. It is completely gluten-free and unlike many of the other "gluten-free" brands, it retains an excellent texture after boiling.

Ancient Harvest's Quinoa Pasta (www.quinoa.com) contains corn, which gives it a bright-yellow color and a good, firm texture.

I also love Japanese soba noodles, which are typically made from buckwheat and can be found in health food stores or the Asian section of your local grocery store. I often use these noodles in stir-fries and salads.

CEREALS

Be especially wary of cereal labeling. The claims often verge on the ridiculous because there are so many labeling loopholes. It's honestly quite hard to find breakfast cereals that don't contain sugar in some form. Evaporated cane juice is an ingredient that you'll see high up on the list. Apart from tasting a little stronger than regular table sugar, there are very few differences. Remember to be suspicious of "made with whole grains" or "zero trans fats," "natural" and "high fiber." These claims mean absolutely nothing. Always read the small print. Finally, be cautious about any of the health claims that any product tries to make. If a cereal is "fortified" with anything, you have to question why it *needs* to be. It's always because the grains have been highly processed and thus stripped of all valuable nutrients.

I recommend the following breakfast cereals for you and your family:

Erewhon cereals (www.usmillsllc.com)
Peace Cereal (www.peacecereal.com)
Nature's Path (www.naturespath.com)
Cascadian Farm (www.cascadianfarm.com)
Archer Farms organic granola cereal (at Target)

My all-time favorite granolas are:

Galaxy Granola, made with apple juice instead of oil, so great for weight loss (www.galaxygranola.com)

Dylan's Chia granolas, made with the super-antioxidant chia seed and so delicious (www.dylanschia.com)

Lessen your eco-impact by purchasing cereal from bulk bins, which you will find at coops, health food stores, and some grocery chains. You can save up to a third on the price and you get less than half the amount of packaging. Oatmeal can be purchased in large cardboard cylindrical containers, and I recommend choosing organic **steel-cut oatmeal** where possible, for it hasn't been stripped of any of the vital nutrients. It takes longer to cook (about twenty minutes) but is well worth the wait. And you can do a bit of kitchen yoga between stirring!

I recommend:

Arrowhead Mills for regular and steel-cut oats (www.arrowheadmills.com)
Bob's Red Mill Organic Scottish Oatmeal www.bobsredmill.com)
Costco's Kirkland Signature Organic brand, available at Costco Stores (www.costco.com)

ECO-IMPACT OF SOY

The Brazilian rain forests are being destroyed to satisfy the enormous global demand for soy. Of soy production worldwide, 85 percent is used for animal feed and biofuels. The farming practices used for soy production on this scale devastate the environment.

Lessen your eco-impact by purchasing organic soy. It's likely that the beans will have been grown in Canada or the United States and will not be genetically modified.

SOY AND SOY-BASED FOODS

As many Gorgeously Green girls are vegetarians or vegans, it's important to look at whether eating soy should be part of your diet plan. Soy contains enzyme inhibitors, which block the action of the very enzymes needed to digest protein. This is why some people get bloated after eating soy. These "antinutrients" are not completely deactivated during cooking. Soy also contains hemagglutinin, a substance that could promote blood clots. Both of these substances are deactivated when soy is fermented, which is why the Japanese almost always eat soy in its fermented form (miso, tempeh, and seitan). Soybeans are also high in phytic acid, which blocks the uptake of essential minerals. However, when soy products are eaten with meat or fish, the phytates are reduced, which is why tofu is mostly eaten in a fish or meat broth in Japan. The isoflavones that are touted as being anticarcinogenic and great for menopausal women are present only in fermented soy products. Suffice it to say, if you enjoy soy, make sure it is always fermented and be really wary of imitation soy meat products, because many of them contain not only soy protein isolate, a highly processed form of soy, but also a host of unhealthy additives, including high-fructose corn syrup. The soy industry has spent billions of dollars touting it as a healthy and perfect food, especially for vegans. But it's a good idea to understand its health implications, especially if you eat a lot of it.

What's the eco-impact of soy foods? Most of the soy grown in the world is genetically modified and farmed intensively, which means massive amounts of fossil fuels and the destruction of biodiversity. Make sure your soy is organic.

The really annoying thing about soy is that it is totally counterproductive if you're trying to lose weight: The isoflavones and phytoestrogens depress thyroid function and thus pack on the pounds. When some women initially switch to a soy-based vegetarian diet, they are thrilled because they lose weight. This is because their poor thyroid is working overtime to counterbalance the effects of the isoflavones—eventually, however, it gives up and these hopeful women wind up regaining their excess weight and then some. Since the Deep Green girl is committed to eating only foods that are completely sustainable, it's annoying because until recently, we thought we'd found the miracle food. Don't despair, though—there's a healthy, eco-friendly way of incorporating delicious fermented soy into many of your dishes (see the recipes section). If you love edamame, always cook them well before serving and make sure they're organic.

I recommend the following fermented soy products:

WestSoy Seitan and WestSoy "Chicken Style" Seitan (www.westsoy.biz)

Lightlife Tempeh (www.lightlife.com)

FISH

I recommend fish on this plan only if it's sustainable, meaning that the variety is not endangered. To find out the best choices for your area, go to www.mbayaq.org and download the appropriate pocket guide. There are quite a few wonderful sustainable whitefish that are readily available: tilapia, halibut, Dover sole, to name a

ECO-IMPACT OF FARMED SHRIMP

Shrimp farming is devastating to the environment. It is damaging because it requires enormous quantities of fish to be caught in the ocean for shrimp feed, most of which is converted to waste that is poured back into the ocean, polluting the water and damaging the mangroves.

Shrimp farming also destroys coastal agriculture because shrimp factories require that seawater be pumped into the man-made freshwater ponds. This causes salinization, which reduces drinking water supplies and destroys nearby crops and trees.

Add to this the thousands of miles that the shrimp have to travel to get to the United States, and your eco-impact is getting pretty high.

few. I will recommend only a few farmed fish on the plan and it will be fish that eat only a vegetarian diet, such as tilapia.

WHAT ABOUT THE CANS?

Make sure you recycle your tuna cans every time, because aluminum can be recycled many times. If I'm using only half a can of tuna, I store the rest in a glass container with a lid. It's a great idea to purchase a set of different size glass bowls with lids for storing leftovers (www.pyrex .com). Remember, certain plastics contain polycarbonate, which has been known to leach the hormone-disrupting chemical bisphenol A (BPA) into your food, so it's better to use glass.

I often get asked about shrimp because they're so popular in the United States. However, the Green Girl needs to think twice because shrimp are largely unsustainable. More than 80 percent of the shrimp we eat in the United States is farmed shrimp from Central America or Asia, where their fish-farming methods devastate the environment. You can eat shrimp with a conscience in the United States now, but you will have to pay more. A fantastic international organization called the Marine Stewardship Council (www.msc.org) has a certification system that encourages sustainable fishing practices. I invite you to look out for the MSC-certified label. The first and only shrimp to get this certification is the Oregon pink shrimp industry. You can buy Oregon pink shrimp in many high-end grocery stores, including Whole Foods. I haven't included shrimp in the eating plan because it can get pretty costly if you are being responsible. I recommend saving shrimp for a very special treat.

I love tuna, always have and always will. It's also a tasty and convenient way to pack protein into salads and sandwiches. However, as we all know, it comes with the mercury price tag, which I'm no longer willing to pay. Fortunately, there are some great low-mercury varieties now available. The most trusted brands are: Wild Planet Tuna (www.1wildplanet.com) and American Tuna (www.americantuna.com). If you are a tuna lover, I suggest buying a couple of cases. It will cost quite a bit more than regular tuna, but I don't think any of you would be too thrilled to get mercury poisoning. Mercury is a neurotoxin, which can cause a variety of debilitating symptoms, depending on the degree of poisoning. I know three women who have mercury poisoning and they suffer from vision, hearing, and speech problems. One of these ladies has difficulty walking, and her speech is slurred. Like most eco-friendly food choices, it's all about moderation: eating the safer foods that we love in moderation so that it works for everyone's budget.

PRODUCE

I include loads of fruits and veggies in your eating plans. To stay within a tight budget, I have specified whether or not it's important to buy organic produce.

Pesticides are used to control all kinds of pests that could destroy a crop. Their use is now so ubiquitous that many crops are becoming pest resistant, which results in the use of even more pesticide. The Environmental Protection Agency has set standards in the United States for the amount and kind of pesticide that is apparently safe for human consumption. These regulations do not take into account that some people eat up to eight servings a day of pesticide-laden fruits and veggies. The limit is apparently safe for a fully grown man, not necessarily a small child. I avoid pesticides whenever I can. If a pesticide can kill an insect or a rodent, it could hurt me, too. Many harmful pesticides that have been banned in the United States still somehow find their way in. And don't forget that imported produce may still be sprayed with these horrific chemicals.

See the list of the most important produce items to buy organic on page 245.

WHAT ABOUT OUR CHILDREN?

A study published by the United States National Research Council (www.nationalacademies.org/nrc) determined that for infants and children, the major source of exposure to pesticides is through diet. A study in 2006 measured the levels of organophosphate pesticide exposure in twenty-three school-age children before and after replacing their diet with organic food. This study found that levels of organophosphate pesticide exposure dropped dramatically and immediately when the children switched to an organic diet. All pesticides are neurotoxins.

Did you know that it's mandatory for every school lunch in Italy to be organic? They really have their priorities straight.

FROZEN FOODS

I'm not a huge fan of the frozen food case because most of the foods displayed are heavily processed and have way too much packaging for a Green Girl. However, buying frozen organic produce is a great option when you can no longer find the fruits and veggies you want in season. In the winter, I always buy a few bags of frozen organic berries to make smoothies with and a few bags of green beans and corn. I would rather have the frozen organic food than fresh nonorganic. Also, as the produce is frozen at its ripest, the freezing will actually keep more nutrients intact than if it sat for weeks in transit unfrozen. The freezing process is energy intensive, for sure; however, we need to compromise here and there to have something delicious and healthful out of season:

www.cascadianfarm.com has a great selection of organic frozen veggies.
www.amyskitchen.com has a great selection of frozen foods.

CONDIMENTS, HERBS, AND SPICES

You'll need to have a really well-stocked spice and herb cupboard for the diet plans.
Look carefully at the following list and make sure you have everything you need.

Bay leaves
Celery salt
Chili powder
Cinnamon
Cumin
Cumin seeds
Curry powder
Dill

EVERYDAY HERB GARDEN

Fresh herbs can transform any dish into a culinary wonder. You'll notice that
I've included a lot of fresh herbs in all the diet plans. They taste wonderful
and are packed with nutrients. To save money, I highly recommend growing
your own. It's so easy.

- If you live in an apartment, get a small window box or four or five mini-
  planters to put on a sunny windowsill.
- If you have a little outdoor space, consider a larger planter or tub that is
  near your kitchen.
- Go to your nearest garden center or nursery and purchase seedlings of
  the following herbs, since they're easier to manage than seeds: parsley,
  cilantro, mint, oregano, rosemary, sage, thyme, and basil.
- You may be able to grow **rosemary**, **parsley**, and mint year-round.
  Make sure you plant mint in its own separate planter, as it will take over
  the entire container and strangle or cover the other herbs.
- In the sunnier months, make sure you plant enough **basil** and **cilantro.**
  You'll likely use a lot of it in summer salads, pastas, salsas, and dips.

Ground red chili pepper
Nutmeg
Oregano
Paprika
Red chili flakes
Tarragon
Thyme
Turmeric
Vanilla essence

The following condiments will also be needed for your plans:

The Wizard's Vegan Worcestershire Sauce★ (www.edwardandsons.com)
Thai fish sauce (www.worldpantry.com)
Hoisin sauce (www.edwardandsons.com)
Organic tomato ketchup

★Avoid regular Worcestershire sauce, as it contains high-fructose corn syrup.

GOOD-FOR-YOU TREATS

My three favorite chocolate companies are: Sjaak's (www.sjaaks.com). This
     family-owned company makes the best mint chocolate I have ever tasted.
Theo Chocolate (www.theochocolate.com). This is the best premium or-
     ganic and fair trade chocolate, ever.
Dagoba Chocolate (www.dagobachocolate.com) is an absolute treat.
Also look for organic, dark, store-brand chocolate. Try to buy chocolate with
     a 70 percent or higher cocoa content.
Cookies and muffins: I love Andean Dream Quinoa Cookies, which come
     in three different flavors (www.andeandream.com).
Fiber cakes are sweet, yummy, and good for you (www.zenbakery.com).

Shopping Tips for the Eating Plans
• Try to do a big shop on the weekend for everything you need for week
     one. Before you go to the store, make sure you have everything you
     need on your list; one large shopping trip saves many high-eco-impact

THREE LOW ECO-IMPACT CHOICES AT A GLANCE!

Milk

1. Raw (glass bottle)
2. Organic unhomogenized (glass bottle)
3. Organic (glass bottle)

Eco-benefit: You will save on the waxed milk cartons that cannot be recycled in most cities. You will be voting with your dollars for healthy milk produced without growth hormones.

Eggs

1. Certified organic (with DHA or omega-3s)
2. Certified humane
3. Cage-free

Eco-benefit: You will be supporting chicken farms that *don't* engage in cruel/inhumane treatment of birds. You will be protecting your health (and the planet) from the devastating effects of heavy pesticide use.

Yogurt

1. Homemade, plain (made with organic whole milk)
2. Organic, plain, whole milk (large tub)
3. Plain, whole milk (large tub)

Eco-benefit: You will be saving on plastic packaging by making your own or using the larger tubs, which last longer.

Bread

1. Organic, sprouted grain
2. 100-percent whole wheat, organic
3. 100-percent whole wheat (no high-fructose corn syrup)

Eco-benefit: You are voting with your dollars for organic farming.

Meat

1. USDA certified organic
2. Grass-fed from a reputable producer
3. Label stating "no hormones administered"

Eco-benefit: You are no longer supporting the devastating effects of intensive factory farming.

Cooking oils

1. Expeller-pressed grape seed oil
2. Virgin coconut oil
3. Pure olive oil

Eco-benefit: You will be supporting the wonderful organic coconut industry. You will be using oils processed without solvents and chemicals that are bad for the environment.

Eating oils (for dressing salads, veggies, etc.)

1. Extra-virgin olive oil (organic)
2. Virgin coconut oil
3. Sesame oil (organic)

Eco-benefit: You will be supporting the growing/farming of organic olives and sesame seeds.

Cereals

1. Nutty Granola (page 267).
2. 100-percent organic (bulk bins)
3. 100-percent organic, whole grains or steel-cut oats

Eco-benefit: You are helping to protect yourself, your family, and the land from the dangerous effects of pesticide residue, and you are saving on packaging and cost by buying in bulk or making your own.

Orange juice

1. Frozen organic
2. Organic in large plastic jug
3. Organic in large waxed carton

Eco-benefit: You are keeping small plastic bottles and waxed milk cartons out of the landfills.

Sweeteners

1. Stevia
2. Honey
3. Maple syrup

Eco-benefit: A little stevia goes a long way—you will typically use a small pinch for a cup of tea or coffee, so a small container will last you a long time, reducing your need to buy plastic containers so often.

small shopping trips later in the week. Go to www.gorgeouslygreen .com/diet to download a printable version of your shopping list.

- The most proven way to avoid wasting food is to make a list and stick to your list. Americans typically throw away 14–20 percent of their food, so let's get thrifty!

- Don't forget to download and print all the coupons you can from www .gorgeouslygreen.com/coupons

- Make sure to take enough reusable bags with you. I typically need five or six ChicoBags for my weekly shop. ChicoBags are extremely durable shopping totes that fold back into a tiny pouch. www.gorgeouslygreen .com/catalog

- Try to go as early as you can in the morning, before the store gets too crowded and it's easier to concentrate.

- Check that you have all the condiments, spices, and herbs listed on pages 56–57, and add whatever is missing to your list.

- When you return from the store, make sure you put your ChicoBags back in your purse and save all the plastic produce bags for your next shop. You can roll them all together and tie them in a loose knot.

- Add three or four pieces of seasonal fruit to your list (pears, plums, peaches, etc.).

- If you know that some of the items on your list may not be available in your local store, check the Web sites that I have provided for store loca-tors or information about how you can buy online.

- Make sure you freeze whatever perishable items you know you won't be eating within two days.

CHAPTER SIX

The Eating Plans

LIGHT GREEN EATING PLAN

This eating plan is the entry level for those of you who care about your health and the planet but who need a bit of a boost to get going. If you follow this plan, you will be lightening your eco-impact by at least 50 percent. You will be cutting down on your meat consumption, making some new organic choices, and learning how to be a little more eco-conscious on a daily basis.

Many of the foods that I have included may be new to you, so take your time to go through the eating plan carefully. I have given you "seasonal options" because eating out of season defeats the purpose of the plan. Remember, eating seasonal and locally produced foods will also be kinder to your pocketbook.

The plan may include more food than you are used to eating on a diet. These are wonderful whole foods that not only will satisfy you but also will keep you glowing and vibrant. I never want you to go hungry, for this will only encourage you to overeat at your next meal. So enjoy the snacks.

Remember, the optimal way to fire up your metabolism is to get moving, and I mean really moving. If you can get in a brisk walk or run before breakfast, you'll be golden. Regardless of your exercise regime (see Section Five: Fitness), it will behoove you to get in another brisk walk before lunch and dinner, too. Whether you work in an office or live in the rolling hills of Virginia, a fast-paced 10–20 minute walk is always possible. It's easier to exercise than to diet, so find a walking buddy now!

If there are days that you can't get out and exercise at all, just cut out the snacks and you'll be good to go. A cup of warming herbal tea is a great substitute in the winter, and an eight-ounce glass of water with the juice of half a lemon works in the summer.

If you don't like any of the meals, simply substitute one of the recipes (see pages 263–330). There are many to choose from.

Finally, you should try to leave about three hours between snacks and meals, so if you get up late one morning or decide to have an early dinner, just cut out the snack.

OG: Look for these letters for the office girl option.

WEEK ONE

Day One:

BEFORE BREAKFAST:
8-ounce glass lemon water (water with juice of half a lemon)

This is an every-morning routine because lemon juice cleanses and stimulates the liver and kidneys and raises the alkalinity of regular water.

BREAKFAST:
½ cup rolled oats (uncooked) with a little rice or almond milk, ½ sliced banana, 1 tsp shredded coconut, and 1 tsp honey

Tea or coffee with your creamer of choice

If you are out and about for breakfast, you can take a packet of instant oatmeal, a yogurt, and a banana with you to work. However, instant oatmeal is a processed food. The oat bran has been removed, leaving a product that is devoid of many of the vitamins and fiber in rolled oats. So if you have to buy instant, get the best-quality organic brand you can find. Try to avoid the extra packaging of single-serving packets.

For the working-away-from-home girl, take your snacks with you in small reusable containers. Also, prepare your salad bright and early and put it in a large reusable container with the dressing on the side (in a small reusable screw-cap jar). If you go to the same office daily, I suggest keeping your dressing in the office fridge. It might be time to invest in a pretty, insulated lunchbox.

MIDMORNING SNACK:
1 apple, peeled or sliced into ½ cup plain yogurt

LUNCH:

Huge salad (as big as you want) made with romaine lettuce (organic and *not* bagged), celery, carrots, cucumber, avocado, sprouts, black olives, 1 hard-boiled egg (or cubed baked tofu), and a small handful of raw almonds

MIDAFTERNOON SNACK:

Smoothie made with 8 ounces of almond milk, ½ cup berries, 1 scoop whey protein powder, 1 tsp honey, and if you want an extra healthy drink, add a scoop of green superfoods (see page 46)

Iced or hot green tea

OG tip: *Quick Protein Shake.* Purchase a blender cup made of BPA-free plastic from www.biossential.com. Keep a carton of rice or almond milk in the office fridge and a container of whey protein powder. This way you can whip up a quick shake without an electric blender. Use 8 ounces of rice or almond milk and 2 scoops of a recommended protein powder (page 46).

Gorgeously Green Dressing

Make a jar of this dressing and keep it in your refrigerator at home or at work. It will last for up to two weeks, so double the recipe if you plan to eat a lot of salad.

1 cup cold-pressed extra-virgin olive oil
½ cup organic apple cider vinegar
1 tsp Dijon mustard
1 tsp honey
1 large clove garlic, crushed
Salt and freshly ground black pepper to taste
Shake all the ingredients in a screw-top jar to emulsify.

DINNER:

1 large portobello mushroom per person: Slice the mushrooms and sauté in 1 tbsp butter and 1 tsp olive oil. Add to the skillet 1 tbsp of soy sauce, 1 tbsp of Worcestershire sauce, and 1 crushed clove of garlic, then cover the pan and fry gently for 5–6 minutes. Add a handful of your favorite cheese (feta, grated cheddar, etc.), and sauté for another 2 minutes. Season with sea salt and pepper. Remove from pan and sprinkle with a generous handful of chopped flat-leaf parsley.

2 cups wilted spinach with a little olive oil and a crushed clove of garlic

1 baked sweet potato or yam with 1 tsp plain yogurt and 1 tsp chopped chives

1 cup organic mint tea sweetened with honey

Day Two:

BEFORE BREAKFAST:

8-ounce glass lemon water (water with juice of half a lemon)

BREAKFAST:

1 poached egg and 1 slice organic whole-wheat or sprouted-grain toast with butter

½ cup plain yogurt with ½ sliced banana

Tea or coffee

OG option: If you are too rushed to poach an egg, have 1 cup of yogurt sprinkled with 1 heaping tbsp of Kashi Go Lean cereal.

> ### TIP
>
> At the beginning of the week, peel and chop 5 or 6 medium carrots into sticks and keep in a resusable container in your fridge.

MIDMORNING SNACK:

3 tbsp White Bean Hummus (page 291) with 1 cup carrot sticks

OG option: You can buy a container of organic hummus and a small bag of peeled organic carrots and keep them in the office refrigerator.

LUNCH:

A bowl of cut-up romaine lettuce sprinkled with 6 raw almonds, ½ cup crumbled feta cheeese, and 5 sliced dried apricots or figs

Add ½ can low-mercury tuna mixed with lemon juice and 2 tsp plain yogurt (or substitute with wild Alaskan salmon)

Dress with Gorgeously Green Dressing (page 63)

MIDAFTERNOON SNACK:

2 sticks celery filled with 1 tbsp almond butter

1 large mug organic green tea

OG tip: Keep a jar of almond butter at your desk. You can spread it on the recommended crackers, celery, or fruit.

DINNER:

Tilapia, Dover sole, or a sustainable whitefish (see page 53, "Fish"): For 2 servings. Heat 2 tsp butter and 1 tbsp olive oil in a skillet. When hot, add fish (½ pound per person) and cook for 3 minutes. Flip the fish and add 1 tbsp capers and ½ cup white wine. Cook for another 3 minutes. Remove the fish from the pan and place on warm plates. Pour the wine-butter sauce over the fish and sprinkle with a handful of chopped flat-leaf parsley.

Eco-tip: Buy salmon only if you can find wild Alaskan summer (frozen is fine). If it's out of season, tilapia, Dover sole, or catfish are kinder on the environment and your wallet than are many other choices.

Steamed broccoli (as much as you want) dressed with a little olive oil and lemon juice

½ cup cooked organic brown rice with a dash of soy sauce. **Cook Once, Eat Twice.**

1 large mug organic mint tea

1 ounce (typically 3 small squares) organic dark chocolate

> ### TIP: COOK ONCE, EAT TWICE
>
> Cook double the amount of rice you will need so you can use leftovers tomorrow. Also use this technique to make double quantities of soup and freeze half for next week.

Day Three:

BEFORE BREAKFAST:

8-ounce glass lemon water (water with juice of half a lemon)

> ### FISHY TIP
>
> Don't forget to visit www.mbayaq.org to find out the most eco-friendly fish choice for your region.

BREAKFAST:

½ cup uncooked rolled oats with ½ sliced apple and 4 chopped walnut halves; stir in ½ cup almond milk and leave to soak for 5 minutes. Sweeten with a little honey.

Tea or coffee with creamer/sweetener of choice

OG option: 2 slices whole-wheat or sprouted-grain toast with almond butter

MIDMORNING SNACK:

1 cup mixed berries with ½ cup cottage cheese or plain yogurt spinkled with shredded coconut (if berries aren't in season, substitute pear or melon)

OG option: 8-ounce glass of Quick Protein Shake (page 63)

LUNCH:

Tabbouleh: 1 cup cooked whole wheat couscous. Place in a bowl with a cut-up tomato, ½ cup chopped flat-leaf parsley, a few chopped mint leaves, 1 tbsp pine nuts (lightly toasted), and 8 sliced black olives.

Serve with ½ ripe avocado with a squeeze of lemon juice and dress with Gorgeously Green Dressing (page 63).

OG option: The office girl can usually find a good couscous salad in the deli. However, this salad is easy enough to make the night before and store in your reusable container.

MIDAFTERNOON SNACK:

8 raw almonds and 4 dried prunes

Iced or hot green tea

DINNER:

Turkey Chili (page 315) served with the leftover brown rice from the day
before

½ cup unsweetened applesauce with 2 tbsp yogurt

Organic mint tea with honey

Day Four:

BEFORE BREAKFAST:

8-ounce glass lemon water (water with juice of half a lemon)

BREAKFAST:

Omelet: 2 eggs with a little goat or feta cheese and broccoli or spinach
(whatever leftover veggies you have)

½ avocado

Vegan option: 1 Orange Bran Flax Muffin (page 268)

Tea or coffee with cream/sweetener of choice

OG option: If you haven't time to make an omelet, you can substitute with
1 cup granola with plain or low-fat Greek yogurt.

MIDMORNING SNACK:

Smoothie made with 8 ounces almond or rice milk, frozen organic mixed
berries, 1 tbsp shredded coconut, 1 scoop whey protein powder, and
1 tsp honey

OG option: Quick Protein Shake (see page 63)

LUNCH:

Gorgeously Green Vegetable Soup (page 286)

Cook Once, Eat Twice: Make double quantities of this soup and freeze
half for next week.

Mug of organic green tea

OG option: The office girl can make this soup way ahead of time and freeze it in a portable reusable container. Before you go to work, stick it in your bag, and at lunch, find a microwave to heat it.

MIDAFTERNOON SNACK:

3 tbsp hummus with 1 cup carrot sticks or 2 sticks of celery

Iced or hot green tea

DINNER:

Fancy Cheesy Grits with Bacon and Arugula (page 297)

1 orange, peeled, sliced, and sprinkled with un-sweetened shredded coconut

1 ounce organic dark chocolate

1 cup mint tea

ECO-IMPACT OF A MICROWAVE OVEN

- Although I'm not a huge fan of microwaves, they have a low eco-impact because they are very energy efficient, particularly for heating small amounts.
- If you are worried about the radiation, the FDA states that the radiation levels within two inches of your oven are well below harmful standards. And if you stand two feet away, the radiation is barely detectable.
- Never heat your food in plastic in a microwave, because chemicals leach out of the plastic into your food when the plastic gets hot.

Day Five:

BEFORE BREAKFAST:

8-ounce glass lemon water (water with juice of half a lemon)

BREAKFAST:

2 slices whole-grain or sprouted-grain toast with almond butter

1 piece seasonal fruit

Tea or coffee

MIDMORNING SNACK:

½ cup plain yogurt with 3 dried prunes and a sprinkle of cinnamon powder

LUNCH:

Large avocado, tomato, and feta or goat cheese salad dressed with extra virgin olive oil and balsamic vinegar

Serve with one warm whole-wheat pita

OG tip: You can make this salad easily in the morning. Squeeze some lemon juice on it to prevent the avocado from going brown.

MIDAFTERNOON SNACK:

1 Iced Café Latte (page 330)

OG option: Protein shake

DINNER:

Tray-Baked Lamb Chops (page 312)

Steamed cabbage with a pat of butter and plenty of salt and pepper

1 mug mint tea

Day Six:

BEFORE BREAKFAST:

8-ounce glass lemon water (water with juice of half a lemon)

BREAKFAST:

1 cup cooked oatmeal with ½ cup almond milk, 6 raw almonds, 1 tbsp cranberries, 1 tsp shredded coconut. Sweeten with raw honey.

Tea or coffee

OG tip: 1 cup instant organic oatmeal with 6 almonds and a handful of dried cranberries

MIDMORNING SNACK:

½ cup cottage cheese with 1 cup of cut-up melon or pineapple

LUNCH:

Black Bean Soup (page 287) **Cook Once, Eat Twice.**

½ avocado, sliced and dressed with good olive oil and lemon juice

OG tip: As this is such a simple soup to prepare, see if you can carve out a few minutes the night before to make it. While it simmers, you can watch TV.

MIDAFTERNOON SNACK:

1 Iced Café Latte (page 330)

OG tip: Quick Protein Shake (see page 63).

Eco-tip: Remember to buy in bulk so you can save on the amount of plastic going to the landfill.

DINNER:

Whole-wheat penne pasta (2 cups cooked pasta per person) topped with plenty of extra-virgin olive oil, capers, chopped black olives, sun-dried tomatoes, and, if you have it, torn-up fresh basil leaves or arugula leaves.

A bowl of summer berries (if they're not in season, buy frozen organic) topped with 1 tbsp plain yogurt and 1 tsp honey

Mint tea

Day Seven:

BEFORE BREAKFAST:

8-ounce glass lemon water (water with juice of half a lemon)

BREAKFAST:

1 soft-boiled egg and 2 slices whole-wheat or spouted-grain toast

Vegan option: ¾ cup Galaxy Granola

1 piece of fruit

OG tip: If you haven't time to boil eggs in the morning, boil one the night before and eat it sliced on your toast.

MIDMORNING SNACK:

4 dried punes and 8 raw almonds

LUNCH:

Pita pocket: Warm a pita pocket and cut in two. Stuff with romaine lettuce, grated carrot, sliced olives, sprouts, and 3 tbsp hummus.

OG tip: Keep a tub of hummus in the office fridge. Pack a lunch box with the lettuce and veggies in a reusable container. If you go to the deli, ask for a veggie sandwich/wrap with hummus, avocado, and salad (skip the cheese and mayo).

MIDAFTERNOON SNACK:

3 tbsp cottage cheese with 1 cup cut-up pineapple or melon

Iced or hot green tea

DINNER:

Roast chicken (1 small organic frying chicken): Slather your chicken with pure olive oil or 2 tbsp melted butter, salt, and pepper, and stuff it with half a lemon. When the chicken is halfway through cooking time (it should take an hour at 400°F for a medium chicken), add some cut-up carrots and potatoes to the baking dish. After roasting, if you are super-concerned about weight, remove the skin.

Cook Once, Eat Twice: Eat only half the chicken if there are two of you, or the whole chicken if there are four of you, and eat the remainder the next night. If there are four or five of you—put in another small chicken for the following night. The idea is that we are saving time and energy here!

Serve with cooked English peas.

1 ounce dark organic chocolate

Mug of mint tea with honey

MAKING SOME STOCK NOW!

Whenever I cook a chicken, I always make some stock with the carcass. It'll lower your eco-impact because you won't need to buy stock/broth in boxes anymore.

Simply put the chicken carcass in a large stockpot with an onion (peeled and chopped), a stalk of celery, a carrot, a bay leaf, and some salt and pepper. Add 6 cups filtered water and simmer over low heat for a couple of hours.

Pour the stock into a glass measuring jug and put in fridge overnight. The next day, skim the layer of fat off the top and pour the stock into an ice cube tray or a glass container to freeze. I love having the ice-cube-size stock cubes at the ready for steam-frying.

(Keep in mind you'll need 6 cups of chicken stock for the Mushroom Risotto on day 7 of week 2.)

WEEK TWO

Day One:

BEFORE BREAKFAST:

8-ounce glass lemon water (water with juice of half a lemon)

BREAKFAST:

If you haven't time to cook these pancakes in the morning, you may want to switch with a weekend breakfast. You can also make the batter the night before.

2 Coconut Protein Pancakes (page 268):

Coffee or tea

MIDMORNING SNACK:

Mango or papaya smoothie (see page 265). Peel and cut up fruit into cubes. Place in blender with 4 ounces almond milk and ½ cup crushed ice. Blend until smooth.

LUNCH:

Salad of cut-up tomatoes, cucumber, black olives, chunks of feta, ½ can tuna or salmon (optional)

MIDAFTERNOON SNACK:

5 Kashi TLC crackers spread with apple butter

Warm or iced green tea

DINNER:

Thai Chicken Salad (page 278) made with chicken left over from the night before

1 cup unsweetened applesauce with 1 tbsp yogurt and 1 tsp honey

Day Two:

BEFORE BREAKFAST:

8-ounce glass lemon water (water with juice of half a lemon)

BREAKFAST:

¾ cup Nutty Granola (page 267), Galaxy Granola, or a Dylan's Chia granola with your choice of milk and ½ sliced banana

Tea or coffee

MIDMORNING SNACK:

Smoothie made with 8 ounces almond milk, a handful of frozen berries, 1 scoop whey protein powder, 1 tsp flaxseed oil, and 1 tsp honey

OG option: 8 oz Protein Shake (page 63)

LUNCH:

Spinach Tortilla (page 295)

Vegan option: Green Lentil Salad (page 276)

OG tip: You can make the tortilla before work, as it's delicious cold, or if you're pressed for time, have a salad with a hard-boiled egg.

MIDAFTERNOON SNACK:

8 raw almonds and 5 dried apricots or figs

Glass of iced tea

DINNER:

Veggie Burgers (page 312)

Salad of 1 cup baby spinach, ½ sliced avocado, and 1 tbsp cranberries dressed with Gorgeously Green Dressing (page 63)

½ papaya with a squeeze of lemon or lime, or a bowl of seasonal berries

Day Three:

BEFORE BREAKFAST:

8-ounce glass lemon water (water with juice of half a lemon)

BREAKFAST:

2 scrambled eggs with 1 tbsp cottage cheese and 1 tsp chopped chives

1 slice whole-wheat toast

Vegan option: ½ cup oatmeal with 1 scoop whey protein powder, ½ sliced banana, and a sprinkling of cinnamon

Tea or coffee

MIDMORNING SNACK:

½ cup yogurt with 1 tsp honey

LUNCH:

Waldorf Salad (page 270) with 1 warm whole-wheat pita

MIDAFTERNOON SNACK:

1 slice sprouted-grain toast with a little peanut butter

OG option: One of the GG-recommended protein bars (pages 45–46)

DINNER:

Tuscan Chicken Stew (page 153)

1 ounce dark chocolate

Mug of mint tea

Day Four:

BEFORE BREAKFAST:

8-ounce glass lemon water (water with juice of half a lemon)

BREAKFAST:

½ cup uncooked rolled oats with 1 sliced apple, 3 chopped dried prunes, and your choice of milk. (Leave to soak for 5 minutes.)

Tea or coffee

MIDMORNING SNACK:

Anything you want—an almond croissant, corn muffin—it's your treat, so go for it!

LUNCH:

Tabbouleh (page 282) with 1 tbsp hummus and 1 whole-wheat pita

Mug of mint tea

OG tip: This salad will take five minutes to prepare the night before. If you can't do it, you can normally buy a decent tabbouleh salad from a deli.

MIDAFTERNOON SNACK:

1 cup cubed cantaloupe or pineapple with 8 raw almonds

DINNER:

Oven-Roasted Florentine Peppers (page 302)

Serve with 1 slice crusty ciabatta or olive bread. Cut off 1 generous slice per person and freeze the rest so you won't be tempted to eat more. Splash out and buy the very best bread you can find since you won't be eating very much bread on this diet. Enjoy every morsel of it. The bread is a must for this recipe because it soaks up the yummy juices after you've eaten up the peppers.

If bell peppers are not in season, make Cozy Cottage Pie (page 323)

A piece of seasonal fruit

Mug of mint tea

Day Five:

BEFORE BREAKFAST:

8-ounce glass lemon water (water with juice of half a lemon)

BREAKFAST:

¾ cup Nutty Granola (page 267), Galaxy Granola, or a Dylan's Chia granola with your choice of milk and ½ sliced banana

OG option: 2 slices whole-wheat toast with almond butter

MIDMORNING SNACK:

Handful of raspberries or blueberries if in season, or a cut-up apple, and ½ cup of cottage cheese

LUNCH:

Corn and Black Bean Salad (page 272)

MIDAFTERNOON SNACK:

5 Kashi TLC crackers with apple butter

DINNER:

Stir-fry ½ cup each of broccoli, carrots, mushrooms, and chopped chard with ½ cup cubed baked tofu or shrimp (6 per person)

1 cup cooked brown rice

1 piece seasonal fruit

Mug of mint tea

Day Six:

BEFORE BREAKFAST:

8-ounce glass lemon water (water with juice of half a lemon)

BREAKFAST:

1 slice whole-wheat or sprouted-grain toast with almond butter and ½ sliced banana

½ cup plain yogurt with 1 tsp honey

Coffee or tea

MIDMORNING SNACK:

2 celery stalks with 1 ounce cheese and 4 black olives

LUNCH:

Coconut Cashew Salad (page 274)

MIDAFTERNOON SNACK:

Fruit smoothie with 8 ounces almond milk, a handful of berries (frozen if not in season), 1 tbsp flaxseed oil, and 1 scoop whey protein powder

DINNER:

Bison/buffalo patties (2 to 4 ounces of meat per person): If you can't get bison, use lean ground beef that is raised without the use of antibiotics or hormones. Grill the patties in a little olive oil with thinly sliced yellow onions.

½ baked sweet potato/yam with 1 tsp plain yogurt and chopped chives

Mixed salad: romaine, sprouts, cucumber, and grated carrot, dressed with Gorgeously Green Dressing (page 63)

A piece of seasonal fruit

Mug of mint tea

Day Seven:

BEFORE BREAKFAST:

8-ounce glass lemon water (water with juice of half a lemon)

BREAKFAST:

2 poached eggs

1 slice whole-wheat or sprouted-grain toast

Vegan option: Substitute eggs with ½ cup oatmeal, 1 scoop whey protein powder, ½ cup berries, and a sprinkle of cinnamon

Coffee or tea

MIDMORNING SNACK:

1 apple and 5 walnut halves

LUNCH:

Gorgeously Green Vegetable Soup (page 286)

MIDAFTERNOON SNACK:

Anything you want—but just *one*! A cookie, a slice of cake, whatever. As it is a treat, don't compromise on quality. The idea is to savor every mouthful.

Iced or hot green tea

DINNER:

    Mushroom Risotto (page 316)

    Green salad (green leaves/spinach, cucumber, celery, herbs. Dress with EVOO
        and lemon juice)

    1 ounce organic dark chocolate

    Mug of mint tea

LIGHT GREEN WEEK ONE SHOPPING LIST

(O) = Try to buy this item organic

Dairy/dairy alternatives/protein

    Creamer of your choice (see GG recommendations)

    1 box almond milk (I like Pacific nut milks [www.pacificfoods.com], and
        any store brand is good.)

    1 box whey protein powder (see GG recommendations, page 45)

    1 dozen cage-free eggs

    1 box butter (from cows not treated with rBGH)

    1 large tub plain or Greek yogurt (Oikos and Fage are great)

    8 ounces feta or goat cheese

    1 large tub cottage cheese **(O)**

    1 can low-mercury tuna (Wild Planet and American Tuna are my favorites)
        or 1 can wild Alaskan salmon

    Tilapia or your choice of a sustainable whitefish (½ pound per person)

    1 whole frying chicken (raised without antibiotics or hormones)

    1½ pounds ground dark turkey breast (raised without antibiotics or hormones)

    1 pound (3 to 4 ounces per person) ground buffalo/bison or beef (raised
        without antibiotics or hormones)

    2 lamb chops (1 per person)

    1 package nitrate-free bacon

Produce

    7 lemons

    2 apples **(O)**

    2 bulbs garlic

Portobello mushrooms (1 per person)

1 bunch flat-leaf parsley

1 bunch fresh cilantro

1 bunch mint leaves

1 bunch basil leaves

1 bunch rosemary

1 large bunch spinach **(O)**

2 yams/sweet potatoes

1 head romaine **(O)**

1 head celery

8 carrots **(O)**

1 cucumber

2 avocados

1 2- to 4-ounce clamshell of sprouts

1 head broccoli

1 small cabbage

2 tomatoes **(O)**

1 orange

1 mango or papaya (can be frozen)

1 melon or pineapple

2 potatoes **(O)**

1 bag frozen mixed berries **(O)**

1 bag frozen English peas **(O)**

1 bag frozen corn **(O)**

1 bag frozen edamame **(O)**

2 yellow onions

1 zucchini

1 bunch chard

8 ounces brown mushrooms

2 jalapeños

1 small cauliflower

4 shallots

1 bag arugula

Oil/vinegar/nuts/seeds

1 16-ounce bag raw almonds★

1 16-ounce bag raw walnuts★

1 16-ounce bag pine nuts

1 bottle extra-virgin olive oil

1 bottle pure olive oil or canola oil

1 bottle apple cider vinegar

1 bottle balsamic vinegar

1 jar Dijon mustard

1 jar honey

1 jar almond butter **(O)**

★Raw nuts are nuts that have not been roasted or salted

Cereals/grains

1 large container rolled oats (Quaker, Wild Harvest, Kirkland, and Country Choice are all great brands.) **(O)**

1 loaf whole-wheat or sprouted-wheat bread (Food for Life at www.foodforlife.com is my favorite brand.)

1 small loaf sourdough bread

1 16-ounce bag brown rice **(O)**

1 box whole-wheat couscous

1 pack whole-wheat pita bread

1 bag Galaxy Granola (or one of the GG-recommended granolas, page 51)

1 bag pearl barley

1 box grits

Extras

Tea or coffee **(O)**

Mint tea and green tea

1 tub hummus

1 jar pitted Kalamata olives

1 jar capers

1 jar sun-dried tomatoes

1 16-ounce bag dried apricots

1 16-ounce bag dried prunes

2 cans black beans

1 16-ounce can whole tomatoes (O)

2 boxes vegetable broth or 1 box bouillon cubes

1 box chicken broth or 1 box bouillon cubes

1 large jar unsweetened applesauce (O)

1 bar dark chocolate

1 jar green superfoods (www.amazinggrass.com; I love Amazing Grass chocolate flavor)

LIGHT GREEN WEEK TWO SHOPPING LIST

Dairy/dairy alternatives/protein

1 4-ounce can of tuna (optional)

1 8-ounce packet of tempeh or extra-firm tofu

4 ounces ground beef/turkey per person

1 16-ounce bag of frozen shrimp

3–4 ounces ground bison/beef per person

4 ounces sliced turkey (nitrate-free)

Produce

4 apples

4 tomatoes

2 cucumbers

1 yellow onion

1 red onion

1 yam

1 lime

1 thumb-size root of ginger

1 bunch spinach

1 ripe avocado

1 zucchini

3 large carrots

1 head of celery

1 head of romaine lettuce

1 head of broccoli

1 handful of green beans (1 16-ounce bag if not in season)

1 green chili pepper

4 ounces white or brown mushrooms

1 1-ounce packet of mixed dried mushrooms

1 head of radishes

1 bunch of fresh cilantro

1 bunch of fresh flat-leaf parsley

1 bunch of fresh basil

1 banana

1 orange

1 16-ounce bag of frozen edamame beans

1 red bell pepper (per person)

1 16-ounce bag of frozen corn or 2 ears of fresh corn

Cereals/grains/pasta/rice

1 box of Kashi TLC crackers

1 box of risotto/arborio rice

1 loaf of ciabatta bread (from bakery in grocery store)

Extras

- 1 bag coconut shreds
- 1 jar apple butter
- 1 bottle of Thai fish sauce (Asian aisle of grocery store)
- 1 bag of dried cranberries
- 1 16-ounce can of garbanzo beans
- 3 16-ounce cans of black beans
- 1 box organic corn tostados
- 1 32-fluid-ounce carton of vegetable broth (or 1 box of vegetable bouillon cubes)
- 1 32-fluid-ounce carton of chicken broth (or 1 box of chicken bouillon cubes)

BRIGHT GREEN EATING PLAN

As you're pretty eco-friendly already, you'll probably be well versed in most of the foods that I recommend on the plan. If you stick to my recommendations, you will be lessening your eco-impact by 75 percent.

I suggest going through the plan very carefully before you begin, making sure that you pick the seasonal options that work for your region.

As in the other plans, I also recommend that you take your daily exercise in small increments because this approach works for anyone, regardless of their circumstances. A brisk 10-minute walk before breakfast and lunch will work even if you are in an office from dawn to dusk. Remember that exercise (and I mean the kind of walking that gets your heart beating) not only stimulates your metabolism but also staves off hunger.

I have created a shopping list for each week. Make sure your list reflects any substitutions you have made.

Day One:

BEFORE BREAKFAST:

8-ounce glass lemon water (add the juice of ½ lemon to filtered water)

This is an every-morning routine because lemon juice cleanses and stimulates the liver and kidneys and raises the alkalinity of regular water.

Tip: You can add 2 ounces of organic aloe vera juice to your lemon water for an extra health boost. Aloe vera juice boasts a number of health benefits: great for digestion, immune system, oral health, and prevention of constipation.

BREAKFAST:

1 bowl steel-cut oatmeal with a little almond milk, 1 tsp shredded coconut, a handful of chopped walnuts, and 1 tsp raw honey

OG option: You can take a packet of instant oatmeal, a yogurt, and a banana with you to work. However, instant oatmeal is a processed food in that the oat bran has been removed, leaving a product devoid of many of the vitamins and fiber in rolled oats—so if you have to buy instant, get the best-quality organic brand you can find.

Tea or coffee with a GG-recommended sweetener and creamer (pages 46 and 37)

MIDMORNING SNACK:

4 dried prunes and a 6-ounce glass of kefir

OG tip: Take your snacks with you in a reusable lunch box (you'll need to invest in some reusable little containers). Also, prepare your salad bright and early and put it in a large reusable container with the dressing on the side (small reusable screw-cap jar). If you go to the same office daily, I suggest keeping your dressing in the office fridge.

LUNCH:

Huge salad (as big as you want) made with romaine lettuce (organic, *not* bagged), celery, carrots, cucumber, avocado, sprouts, radishes, black olives, a hard-boiled egg, and a small handful of raw almonds dressed with Gorgeously Green Dressing (see page 63)

MIDAFTERNOON SNACK:

1 slice sprouted-grain toast, spread with a little apple butter

1 mug organic green tea, sweetened with honey or stevia. Can be served hot or iced.

OG option: GG-recommended protein bar (pages 45–46)

DINNER:

1 large portobello mushroom (per person), sliced and sautéed in a little olive oil, 1 tbsp Worcestershire sauce, 1 tbsp soy sauce, and 1 crushed clove of garlic. Season with salt and pepper and sprinkle after cooking with a generous handful of chopped flat-leaf parsley.

2 cups wilted spinach with a little olive oil and 1 crushed clove of garlic

1 baked sweet potato/yam with 1 tsp sour cream or plain yogurt and
   chives

1 ounce (about 3 small squares) organic dark chocolate

Mint tea sweetened with honey

Day Two:

BEFORE BREAKFAST:

8-ounce glass lemon water (add the juice of ½ lemon to filtered water)

BREAKFAST:

2 poached eggs

1 slice sprouted-grain toast with butter

Vegan option: Substitute eggs with 1 cup oatmeal, 1 scoop whey protein
   powder, ½ cup mixed berries, 1 tsp honey, and a sprinkle of cinnamon.

Tea or coffee

MIDMORNING SNACK:

5 walnut halves and 1 piece seasonal fruit

LUNCH:

Gorgeously Green Wrap: Fill a gently warmed sprouted-grain tortilla with
   baby spinach, sliced avocado, sliced olives, sliced red bell peppers (if bell
   peppers aren't in season, use a jar of marinated bell peppers instead), and
   3 tbsp hummus

OG tip: You can make this wrap before you go to work or you can order a
   veggie and hummus wrap from your local deli.

MIDAFTERNOON SNACK:

2 stalks celery filled with 1 tbsp almond butter

1 mug or glass of green tea

OG tip: Keep a jar of almond butter at your desk. You can spread it on the
   recommended crackers, celery, or fruit.

DINNER:

Tilapia or Dover sole (½ pound per person): For two people. Put 2 tsp butter
   and 1 tsp olive oil in a skillet on medium heat. When hot, add the fish and

cook for 3 minutes on one side. Flip it over and add 1 tbsp capers, ½ cup white wine, salt, and pepper Cook for another 3 minutes, until cooked through. Remove fish and put on the warmed plates. Pour over the sauce from the pan and sprinkle with a handful of chopped flat-leaf parsley.

As much steamed broccoli as you want (dress it with a little olive oil and lemon juice)

½ cup cooked organic brown rice with a dash of soy sauce. **Cook Once, Eat Twice.**

½ cup Greek yogurt with 4 raw almonds and 1 tsp honey

Mint tea sweetened with honey

Day Three:

BEFORE BREAKFAST:

8-ounce glass lemon water (add the juice of ½ lemon to filtered water)

BREAKFAST:

½ cup uncooked rolled oats with 1 sliced apple and 5 walnut halves. Stir in a little almond milk and leave to soak for 5 minutes. Sweeten with a little honey.

1 slice sprouted-grain toast with almond butter. (If you are away from home and cannot get sprouted-grain toast, substitute with whole-grain toast.)

Tea or coffee

MIDMORNING SNACK:

3 tbsp White Bean Hummus (page 291) with raw veggies

OG tip: It's also a great idea to keep a tub of organic hummus and a reusable container of raw veggies (such as cut-up carrots or celery) in your office fridge.

LUNCH:

A bowl of cut-up romaine lettuce sprinkled with raw almonds, feta cheese, and 5 sliced dried apricots

Add ½ can low-mercury tuna mixed with lemon juice and 2 tsp Greek yogurt (optional) and dress with Gorgeously Green Dressing (page 63)

MIDAFTERNOON SNACK:

Iced Café Latte (page 330)

or

Mug of green tea

DINNER:

Turkey Chili (page 315) served with the leftover brown rice from the night before

1 cup cherries or 2 plums or 1 sliced pear

Mint tea

Day Four:

BEFORE BREAKFAST:

8-ounce glass lemon water (add the juice of ½ lemon to filtered water)

BREAKFAST:

Omelet: 2 eggs with 1 level tsp goat cheese or feta cheese and broccoli or spinach (add red bell peppers if in season)

½ avocado

1 slice sprouted-grain toast

Vegan option: Substitute eggs with 1 cup cooked oatmeal, 1 scoop whey protein powder, 1 tbsp dried cranberries, handful of chopped walnuts, and 1 tsp honey

Tea or coffee

OG tip: If you haven't time to make an omelet, you can substitute with a fist-size portion of one of the recommended cereals (page 51), almond or rice milk, and ½ banana.

MIDMORNING SNACK:

Smoothie made with 8 ounces almond or rice milk, ½ cup frozen organic blueberries, 1 scoop whey protein powder, 1 tsp flaxseed oil, 1 tsp shredded coconut, and 1 tsp raw honey

OG option: Quick Protein Shake (page 63)

LUNCH:

Gorgeously Green Vegetable Soup (page 286) **Cook Once, Eat Twice**

OG tip: The office girl can make this soup way ahead of time and freeze it in a portable-size reusable container. Before you go to work, stick it in your bag, and then at lunch, find a microwave to heat it.

MIDAFTERNOON SNACK:

½ cup plain yogurt with 4 sliced prunes and a sprinkle of cinnamon
Iced or hot green tea

DINNER:

Coconut Cashew Salad (page 274) (Make more than you need; it keeps beautifully for a few days in an airtight container in your fridge.)
½ cup organic applesauce with 1 tbsp plain yogurt and 1 tsp honey
Mint tea

Day Five:

BEFORE BREAKFAST:

8-ounce glass lemon water (add the juice of ½ lemon to filtered water)

BREAKFAST:

2 slices sprouted-grain toast with almond butter and ½ sliced banana on top
Tea or coffee

MIDMORNING SNACK:

2 tbsp White Bean Hummus (page 291) with raw veggies

LUNCH:

Large salad of avocado, tomato, black olive, and feta cheese dressed with olive oil and balsamic vinegar (if tomatoes aren't in season, substitute with sun-dried tomatoes)
1 piece seasonal fruit
OG tip: You should be able to get this salad in a good deli.

MIDAFTERNOON SNACK:

Smoothie made with 8 ounces rice or almond milk, 1 scoop whey protein powder, 1 tbsp almond butter, 1 tsp unsweetened cocoa powder, and 1 tsp honey
OG option: Quick Protein Shake (page 63)

DINNER:

Cozy Cottage Pie (page 323) **Cook Once, Eat Twice.**

1 ounce organic dark chocolate

Mint tea

Day Six:

BEFORE BREAKFAST:

8-ounce glass lemon water (add the juice of ½ lemon to filtered water)

BREAKFAST:

¾ cup oatmeal with 6 raw almonds, a little rice or almond milk, and ½
   sliced banana, sweetened with honey

Tea or coffee

MIDMORNING SNACK:

8-ounce glass kefir

OG option: GG-recommended protein bar (pages 45–46)

LUNCH:

Leftover Coconut and Cashew Curry Crunch (delicious cold)

MIDAFTERNOON SNACK:

1 serving of any of the recommended crackers (page 49), spread with apple
   butter

Iced or hot green tea

DINNER:

Quinoa pasta (see recommended brands, page 50): This is very high in protein, but it is still a carb, so watch your portion size. Stick to the serving
   suggestions on the box.

Top with plenty of olive oil, capers, chopped-up black olives, sun-dried tomatoes, and, if you have them, torn-up fresh basil leaves.

If they're in season, you can also add fresh tomatoes, and a generous grating
   of fresh Parmesan cheese

A bowl of summer berries if organic and in season. If not, substitute with 1
   cup sliced pear, mango, or melon.

1 orange, peeled and sliced, with 1 tbsp shredded coconut

Mint tea

Day Seven:

BEFORE BREAKFAST:

8-ounce glass lemon water (add the juice of ½ lemon to filtered water)

BREAKFAST:

1 soft-boiled egg

2 slices sprouted-grain toast spread with butter

1 piece of fruit

Vegan option: Substitute egg with ¾ cup oatmeal, 1 scoop whey protein powder, 1 tsp shredded coconut, 5 raw almonds, and 1 tsp honey

Tea or coffee

OG option: If you haven't time to boil eggs this morning, make yourself a quick smoothie with whey protein powder, milk, and banana and or frozen/fresh berries.

MIDMORNING SNACK:

½ cup Greek yogurt with ½ cup mixed berries (seasonal option: 4 sliced dried apricots)

LUNCH:

Green Lentil Salad (page 276) **Cook Once, Eat Twice.**

OG option: You can pick an easier salad from one of the other days or make this incredibly nutritious lentil salad ahead of time. It keeps well for three or four days.

MIDAFTERNOON SNACK:

2 tbsp hummus with raw veggies

Iced or hot green tea

DINNER:

Roast chicken (1 small organic frying chicken): Massage 1 tbsp of butter or 1 tbsp pure olive oil into the skin. Season with salt and pepper, and stuff it with half a lemon. Halfway through cooking time (it should take an hour at 400°F for a medium chicken), cut up some carrots and potatoes into bite-size cubes and add to the baking dish. If you are super-concerned about weight, remove the skin after roasting.

Cook Once, Eat Twice: Eat only half the chicken if there are only two of you and have the remainder the next night. If there are four or five of you—put in another small chicken for the following night. The idea is that we are saving time and energy here!

Serve with cooked peas

1 ounce dark organic chocolate

Mug of mint tea with honey

WEEK TWO

Day One:

BEFORE BREAKFAST:

8-ounce glass lemon water (add the juice of ½ lemon to filtered water)

BREAKFAST:

2 Coconut Protein Pancakes (page 268)

Tea or coffee

If you haven't time to cook these pancakes in the morning, you may want to swap with a weekend breakfast. You can also make the batter the night before so that it's superquick in the morning. If you are wheat-intolerant, replace the wheat germ and whole-wheat flour with almond flour.

MIDMORNING SNACK:

1 apple and 1 tbsp almond butter

LUNCH:

Turkey sandwich made on sprouted-grain bread: nitrate-free sliced turkey, lettuce, tomato, cucumber, sprouts, Dijon mustard, and pickles, with 1 tsp of a GG-recommended mayonnaise (page 341).

OG tip: If you cannot get sprouted-grain bread at the deli, substitute with whole-wheat bread.

MIDAFTERNOON SNACK:

½ cup kefir with 1 cup cubed melon, mango, or pineapple

Iced or hot green tea

DINNER:

Thai Chicken Salad (page 278) made with chicken left over from the night
before

2 squares dark chocolate

Day Two:

BEFORE BREAKFAST:

8-ounce glass lemon water (add the juice of ½ lemon to filtered water)

BREAKFAST:

1 cup Galaxy Granola or Nutty Granola (page 267) with milk of your choice
and ½ sliced banana

MIDMORNING SNACK:

Smoothie made with 8 ounces almond milk, frozen berries, 1 scoop whey
protein, 1 tbsp flaxseed oil, 1 tsp green superfoods powder (see recommended protein powders, page 46), and 1 tsp raw honey

OG option: Quick Protein Shake (page 63)

LUNCH:

Leftover Green Lentil Salad

MIDAFTERNOON SNACK:

8 raw almonds and 4 or 5 apricots or dried prunes

Green tea

DINNER:

Veggie Burgers (page 312)

Serve with a spinach, avocado, and cranberry salad

Papaya, with a squeeze of lemon or lime juice, or a large slice of cantaloupe

Day Three:

BEFORE BREAKFAST:

8-ounce glass lemon water (add the juice of ½ lemon to filtered water)

BREAKFAST:

2 ounces of tempeh or tofu scrambled in 1 tsp olive oil with some finely chopped onion, bell peppers, and zucchini. Serve with 1 slice of sprouted grain toast.

Tea or coffee

OG option: ¾ cup oatmeal with almond milk, ½ sliced banana, and a handful of chopped walnuts

MIDMORNING SNACK:

3 stalks celery and 1 tbsp almond butter

LUNCH:

Large spinach salad with sliced mushrooms, black olives, sprouts, radishes, cucumbers, and cut-up hard-boiled egg or baked tofu dressed with Gorgeously Green Dressing (page 63)

MIDAFTERNOON SNACK:

Mango or papaya smoothie (see page 265): Peel and cut up the fruit into cubes. Place in blender with 4 ounces almond milk and ½ cup crushed ice. Blend until smooth.

OG option: GG-recommended protein bar (pages 45–46)

DINNER:

2 organic corn tostadas per person, filled with ground beef or turkey, black beans, shredded lettuce, chopped tomato, Greek yogurt, and chopped cilantro

1 orange, peeled and sliced, sprinkled with 1 tbsp shredded unsweetened coconut

Mint tea

Day Four:

BEFORE BREAKFAST:

8-ounce glass lemon water (add the juice of ½ lemon to filtered water)

BREAKFAST:

¾ cup steel-cut oatmeal, 1 tbsp almond milk, 1 tsp honey, and 1 tbsp chopped walnuts

Tea or coffee

OG option: Substitute steel-cut oatmeal with regular or instant oatmeal.

MIDMORNING SNACK:

1 cut-up pear or apple with 1 ounce cheese or 6-ounces glass kefir

LUNCH:

Tabbouleh (page 282) with ½ avocado dressed with good olive oil and
lemon juice

OG tip: This salad will take five minutes to prepare the night before. If you
can't do it, you can normally buy a decent tabbouleh salad from a deli.

MIDAFTERNOON SNACK:

Iced Café Latte (page 330)

DINNER:

Oven-Roasted Florentine Peppers (page 302)

Serve with 1 slice crusty ciabatta or olive bread. Cut off 1 generous slice per
person and freeze the rest so you won't be tempted to eat more. Splash
out and buy the very best bread you can find; you won't be eating very
much bread on this diet—so best to enjoy every morsel of it while you
can. The bread is a must for this recipe because it soaks up the yummy
juices when you've eaten up the peppers.

If bell peppers aren't in season, pick a dinner recipe for the appropriate season from Winter Dinners recipes (page 315).

1 Miraculous Chocolate Macaroon (page 177)

Mint tea

Day Five:

BEFORE BREAKFAST:

8-ounce glass lemon water (add the juice of ½ lemon to filtered water)

BREAKFAST:

2 scrambled eggs

1 slice sprouted-grain toast spread with a little butter

Vegan option: ¾ cup cooked quinoa grains topped with 1 cup sautéed
veggies

Coffee or tea

OG option: 2 slices whole-wheat or sprouted-grain toast with almond butter

MIDMORNING SNACK:

Whatever you fancy—almond croissant or pain au chocolate, banana muffin or a lemon slice; just surprise yourself with a delicious treat. The only caveat is that this snack contain no high-fructose corn syrup or partially hydrogenated oils.

LUNCH:

Black Bean Soup (page 287)

MIDAFTERNOON SNACK:

GG-recommended protein bar (pages 45–46)

DINNER:

Stir-Fry: In a wok, heat 1 tsp grape seed oil and 1 tsp toasted sesame oil. Stir-fry broccoli florets, mushrooms, green beans (frozen if not in season), ½ cup boiled edamame, and ½ cup cubed baked tofu or 1 cup shrimp. Sprinkle with low-sodium soy sauce and toasted sesame seeds.

If necessary, substitute with whatever veggies are in season (bell peppers, asparagus, snow peas, etc.).

Serve with ¾ cup cooked soba noodles

1 piece seasonal fruit

Mint tea

Day Six:

BEFORE BREAKFAST:

8-ounce glass lemon water (add the juice of ½ lemon to filtered water)

BREAKFAST:

2 slices sprouted-grain toast, spread with almond butter and ½ sliced banana

MORNING SNACK:

Gorgeously Green Smoothie (page 266)

LUNCH:

Waldorf Salad (page 270)

OG tip: It's easy to make this salad the night before.

MIDAFTERNOON SNACK:

½ cup raw carrots, 2 tbsp hummus, and 4 black olives

Iced or hot green tea

DINNER:

Ground bison/buffalo or ground beef patties (3 to 4 ounces of meat per person) grilled with sliced yellow onions and mushrooms

½ baked yam/sweet potato and 1 tsp plain yogurt and chives

Mixed salad: lettuce, cucumber, sprouts, grated carrots, and olives or Crunchy Watercress Delight (page 271)

1 Miraculous Chocolate Macaroon (page 177)

Mint tea

Day Seven:

BEFORE BREAKFAST:

8-ounce glass lemon water (add the juice of ½ lemon to filtered water)

BREAKFAST:

2 poached eggs

1 slice sprouted-grain toast

OG option: ½ cup Galaxy Granola and ½ cup Greek yogurt

Tea or coffee

Vegan option: 2 slices sprouted-grain toast with almond or peanut butter

MIDMORNING SNACK:

1 apple with 6 raw almonds

LUNCH:

Corn and Black Bean Salad (page 272)

MIDAFTERNOON SNACK:

Pick any cookie or treat from the GG-recommended list (page 57)

DINNER:

Mushroom Risotto (page 316) with green salad

1 piece seasonal fruit

Mint tea

BRIGHT GREEN WEEK ONE SHOPPING LIST

Dairy/dairy alternatives/protein

Creamer of choice

1 carton almond milk (www .pacificfoods.com)

32-ounce bottle organic kefir (see recommended brands, page 37)

1 dozen organic eggs

1 1-pound tub fat-free Greek yogurt

1 16-ounce box butter (from cows not treated with rBST)

1 large tub whey protein powder (Energy First: www.energy firstproteinpowder.com)

8 ounces feta cheese

1 15-ounce tub ricotta cheese

1 small carton buttermilk (from cows not treated with rBST)

1 small hunk Parmesan cheese

Tilapia or Dover sole (½ pound per person)

1 can low-mercury tuna (Wild Planet or American Tuna)

1½ pounds ground dark turkey (organic or hormone- and antibiotic-free)

1 whole frying chicken (organic or hormone- and antibiotic-free)

Produce

7 lemons

5 apples (O)

1 orange

3 bananas

1 head romaine lettuce (O)

1 Napa cabbage

1 bunch chard (O)

1 head celery (O)

8 carrots (O)

1 cucumber (O)

3 avocados

4-ounce package sprouts

1 bunch radishes

2 garlic bulbs

Portobello mushrooms (1 per person)

1 bunch flat-leaf parsley

1 bunch cilantro

1 bunch basil

8 ounces brown mushrooms

2 bunches or bags spinach (O)

4 yams

4 yellow onions (O)

1 piece fresh ginger root (about 2 fingers' worth)

1 parsnip

1 leek

1 medium zucchini

1 large head broccoli

3 avocados

red bell peppers (1 per person) **(O)**

1 small cauliflower

1 ear corn (or one bag frozen corn) **(O)**

1 bag frozen edamame **(O)**

1 bag frozen mixed berries **(O)**

1 bag frozen peas **(O)**

Oil/vinegar/nuts/seeds

16-ounce bag raw almonds

16-ounce bag raw walnuts

16-ounce bag raw cashew nuts

16-ounce bag green lentils

1 jar almond butter **(O)**

1 jar raw honey

Extra-virgin olive oil (cold-pressed)

1 8-ounce bottle flaxseed oil

1 jar virgin coconut oil (www.tropicaltraditions.com)

Organic apple cider vinegar

1 bottle balsamic vinegar

1 jar Dijon mustard

Cereals/grains/pasta

1 30-ounce container steel-cut oats **(O)**

1 30-ounce container rolled oats **(O)**

1 loaf sprouted-grain bread (www.foodforlife.com)

1 package sprouted-grain tortillas (www.foodforlife.com)

1 32-ounce bag brown rice **(O)**

1 32-ounce bag pearl barley

1 box GG-recommended crackers (page 50)

1 8-ounce box Ancient Harvest Quinoa pasta (serves 4)

Extras

Tea or coffee **(O)**

Green and mint tea **(O)**

1 bar dark chocolate **(O and fair-trade)**

1 can unsweetened cocoa powder **(O)**

1 bottle white cooking wine

1 16-ounce bag shredded unsweetened coconut

1 16-ounce bag dried apricots

1 16-ounce bag dried prunes

1 bag raisins **(O)**

1 8-ounce container hummus **(O)**

2 boxes vegetable broth or 1 box vegetable bouillon cubes

1 15-ounce can kidney beans

1 16-ounce can tomatoes

1 6-ounce can tomato paste

1 24-ounce jar unsweetened applesauce **(O)**

1 large jar pitted Kalamata olives

1 small jar capers

1 large jar sun-dried tomatoes

1 large jar marinated bell peppers

BRIGHT GREEN WEEK TWO SHOPPING LIST

Dairy/dairy alternatives/protein

    2 ounces nitrate-free sliced turkey

    Ground bison/buffalo or lean ground beef (raised without antibiotics or hormones) (3 to 4 ounces per person)

    1 8-ounce package tempeh (www.lightlife.com)

    1 8-ounce package baked tofu or ½ pound shrimp

    2 ounces goat cheese

Produce

    2 apples **(O)**

    4 tomatoes

    Papaya or cantaloupe

    1 mango

    1 large bunch or bag spinach **(O)**

    4 ounces white mushrooms

    1 package dried mixed mushrooms

    2 oranges **(O)**

    Red bell peppers (1 per person)

    1 head broccoli

    1 bunch watercress

    1 jicama

    1 red onion

    1 green chile

    1 or 2 jalapeños

    1 lime

    1 bunch scallions

    1 bunch fresh mint

Oils

    1 bottle grape seed oil

    1 bottle toasted sesame oil

    1 bottle peanut oil

    1 small bottle chili oil (optional)

Cereals/grains/pasta/rice
  1 bag Galaxy Granola (or one from recommended list, page 51)
  1 10-ounce package soba noodles
  1 box whole-wheat couscous
  1 box risotto (arborio) rice
  1 box organic tostado shells (www.naturalgrocers.com)

Extras
  1 box organic veggie burgers
  3 15-ounce cans black beans **(O)**
  1 bottle agave syrup
  1 small bottle Thai fish sauce (Asian section of market)
  1 small bag peanuts

DEEP GREEN EATING PLAN

This eating plan is designed to lessen your eco-impact by 95 percent. By choosing the foods on the plan and adhering to the suggestions below, you will be making a huge difference.

Since you are a Deep Green Girl, I invite you to have a look through the suggestions below. Everything I have suggested is great for your health and your pocketbook as well as your considerably improved eco-impact.

- You are going to make your own yogurt for this eating plan. I highly recommend visiting www.lucyskitchenshop.com, where you'll find a fantastic yogurt maker and the starter cultures. The whole lot will cost you less than a pair of jeans and last you a lot longer. A couple of days before you start your eating plan, you will need to make a batch of yogurt.
- Why not also have a go at making your own bread for this plan? You can purchase a new bread maker, which also costs less than a pair of jeans, or get one from a thrift store. The beauty of making your own is that you can make a gluten-free loaf, a vegan loaf, or anything you fancy. If you're a super-crunchy girl, you may decide to make your own bread without a machine.

- You will need to make your own granola for your plan (page 267).
- You can make your own sprouts, too. It takes about a week for them to sprout, so get going the week before you start your plan.
- Try to make your own hummus (page 292). It'll cost a fraction of the price of store-bought hummus and you'll be decreasing your eco-impact by eliminating the plastic tub.
- Since herbs are suggested in many of the recipes on your plan, start a planter, either on a windowsill or just outside your kitchen (page 56).
- Commit to composting all your produce waste. It makes the best and most inexpensive plant fertilizer as well as lessening your eco-impact significantly.

Day One:

BEFORE BREAKFAST:

8-ounce glass lemon water (add the juice of ½ lemon to filtered water)

BREAKFAST:

¾ cup steel-cut oatmeal with a little almond milk, 1 tsp shredded coconut, 1 tsp raw honey, and 1 tbsp chopped walnuts

Steel-cut is the healthiest kind of oatmeal because it hasn't been stripped of anything—it is a whole food.

Tea or coffee

OG tip: You can take a package of organic instant oatmeal, a container of yogurt, and a banana with you to work. However, instant oatmeal is a processed food in that the oat bran has been removed, leaving a product that is devoid of many of the vitamins and fiber in steel-cut oatmeal— so if you have to buy instant, get the best-quality organic brand you can find.

OG tip: Take your snacks with you in a reusable lunch box (you'll need to invest in some small reusable containers). Also, prepare your salad bright and early and put it into a large reusable container with the dressing on the side (small reusable screw-cap jar). If you go to the same office daily, I suggest keeping your dressing in the office fridge.

MIDMORNING SNACK:

1 apple or pear and a 6-ounce glass of kefir

LUNCH:

Huge salad (as big as you want) made with romaine lettuce (organic, *not* bagged), celery, carrots, cucumber, avocado, radishes, black olives, 1 hard-boiled egg, and a small handful of raw almonds, dressed with 1 tbsp Gorgeously Green Dressing (page 63).

MIDAFTERNOON SNACK:

I slice sprouted-grain toast spread with a little apple butter

Hot or iced green tea

OG option: Choose a GG-recommended protein bar (pages 45–46) or make your own ahead of time.

DINNER:

1 large portobello mushroom (per person), sliced and sautéed in a little olive oil with 1 tbsp Worcestershire sauce, 1 tbsp soy sauce, and 1 crushed clove of garlic. Season with salt and pepper and sprinkle with a generous handful of chopped flat-leaf parley.

2 cups wilted spinach with a little olive oil and a crushed clove of garlic

½ baked yam

1 ounce (about 3 small squares) dark chocolate

Mint tea sweetened with honey

Day Two:

BEFORE BREAKFAST:

8-ounce glass lemon water (add the juice of ½ lemon to filtered water)

BREAKFAST:

2 poached eggs

1 slice sprouted-grain toast

Vegan option: ½ cup uncooked rolled oats, ½ cup almond milk, 1 small apple (peeled and sliced), and 4 walnut halves

Tea or coffee

MIDMORNING SNACK:

2 tbsp White Bean Hummus (page 291) with raw veggies

LUNCH:

Salad made of cut-up romaine lettuce and sprouts sprinkled with toasted almonds, feta cheese, and 5 sliced dried apricots

Add ½ can of low-mercury tuna (mixed with lemon juice and 2 tsp plain yogurt) and dress with Gorgeously Green Dressing (page 63).

Vegan option: Cut-up romaine lettuce sprinkled with toasted almonds, sprouts, edamame, garbanzo beans, and 5 sliced apricots, sliced, and dressed with Gorgeously Green Dressing (page 63)

MIDAFTERNOON SNACK:

½ cup homemade yogurt with 3 sliced dried prunes and 1 tsp raw honey

Vegan option: ½ cup soy kefir

Hot or iced green tea

OG tip: Keep a jar of almond butter at your desk. You can spread it on the recommended crackers, celery, or fruit.

DINNER:

Tempeh Hotpot (page 313)

As much steamed broccoli as you want

½ cup steamed brown rice. **Cook Once, Eat Twice.**

Mint tea sweetened with honey

1 ounce organic dark chocolate

Day Three:

BEFORE BREAKFAST:

8-ounce glass lemon water (add the juice of ½ lemon to filtered water)

BREAKFAST:

1 slice homemade whole-wheat or sprouted-grain toast, spread with almond butter and ½ sliced banana (if you are away from home and you cannot get sprouted-grain toast, substitute with whole-grain toast)

Tea or coffee

MIDMORNING SNACK:

Gorgeously Green Smoothie (page 266).

OG tip: Why not invest in an office blender? You'll save not only dollars but also plastic packaging.

LUNCH:

Tabbouleh: Combine 1 cup whole-wheat couscous, 1 cut-up tomato, ½ cup chopped flat-leaf parsley, a few chopped mint leaves, pine nuts, and black olives

Serve with ½ ripe avocado with a squeeze of lemon juice

OG tip: The office girl can usually find a good couscous salad in the deli. However, this salad is easy enough to make the night before and store in your reusable container. If you are intolerant to wheat, replace the couscous with quinoa grains.

MIDAFTERNOON SNACK:

2 tbsp White Bean Hummus (page 291) with 2 stalks celery

Hot or iced tea

DINNER:

Black Bean Soup (page 287) with Crunchy Watercress Delight (page 271)

1 warmed sprouted-grain tortilla

1 cup of cherries or 2 plums (substitute 5 dried apricots or figs if fresh cherries or plums are not in season)

Mint tea

Day Four:

BEFORE BREAKFAST:

8-ounce glass lemon water (add the juice of ½ lemon to filtered water)

BREAKFAST:

Omelet: 2 eggs with a little goat cheese and broccoli or spinach

½ avocado

Vegan option: 1 cup Nutty Granola (page 267) with almond milk

Tea or coffee

OG tip: If you haven't time to make an omelet, you can substitute ¾ cup Nutty granola or Galaxy Granola with almond or rice milk.

MIDMORNING SNACK:

An 8-ounces smoothie made with almond or rice milk, frozen organic blueberries, 1 scoop hemp protein powder, 1 tsp flaxseed oil, and 1 tsp honey

LUNCH:

Gorgeously Green Vegetable Soup (page 286)

Cook Once, Eat Twice: Make double quantities of soup and freeze half for the following week.

OG tip: The office girl can make this soup way ahead of time and freeze it in a portable-size reusable container. Before you go to work, stick it in your bag, and then at lunch, find a microwave to heat it.

MIDAFTERNOON SNACK:

5 walnut halves with a handful of dried cranberries

Hot or iced green tea

DINNER:

Coconut Cashew Salad (page 274). **Cook Once, Eat Twice.**

Serve with ½ cup brown rice (leftover)

½ cup applesauce with 2 tsp plain yogurt or kefir

Mint tea

Day Five:

BEFORE BREAKFAST:

8-ounce glass lemon water (add the juice of ½ lemon to filtered water)

BREAKFAST:

2 slices homemade whole-wheat or sprouted-grain toast with almond butter and ½ sliced banana on top

MIDMORNING SNACK:

1 Coconut, Walnut, and Banana Muffin (page 269)

LUNCH:

Salad made of large avocado, tomato, black olive, and goat cheese dressed with olive oil and balsamic vinegar

Vegan option: Substitute goat cheese with 1 cup garbanzo beans.

1 piece seasonal fruit

MIDAFTERNOON SNACK:

8-ounces smoothie made with rice or almond milk, fresh or frozen organic berries, 1 tsp flaxseed oil, and 1 scoop hemp protein powder

OG option: Quick Protein Shake (page 63)

DINNER:

Cozy Cottage Pie (page 323)

1 ounce organic dark chocolate

Mint tea

Day Six:

BEFORE BREAKFAST:

8-ounce glass lemon water (add the juice of ½ lemon to filtered water)

BREAKFAST:

½ cup oatmeal with 6 or 7 raw almonds, ½ cup plain yogurt or soy kefir, and ½ sliced banana

MIDMORNING SNACK:

1 homemade Crispy Coconut and Flax Protein Bar (page 176)

LUNCH:

Leftover Coconut Cashew Salad (delicious cold)

OG option: Make a salad before you leave with either ½ can tuna, 2 hard-boiled eggs or cut-up tofu, minced red onion, and 1 tsp Spectrum Mayonnaise (Light Canola is best)

MIDAFTERNOON SNACK:

8 raw almonds and 4 dried prunes

Hot or iced green tea

DINNER:

Quinoa pasta (This is very high in protein; however, it is still a carb, so watch your portion size. Stick to the serving suggestions on box. If it says the package serves 4, then take out no more than one quarter for yourself.) Top with plenty of olive oil, capers, chopped-up black olives, and sun-dried tomatoes, and if you have it, torn-up fresh basil leaves. If they are in season, you can also add fresh tomatoes.

A bowl of summer berries (if in season and you can get organic), or slice up a pear, mango, or some melon.

Mint tea

1 orange, peeled and sliced, with 1 tbsp unsweetened shredded coconut

Day Seven:

BEFORE BREAKFAST:

8-ounce glass lemon water (add the juice of ½ lemon to filtered water)

BREAKFAST:

1 soft-boiled egg

2 slices sprouted-grain toast

1 piece seasonal fruit

Vegan option: 1 cup Nutty Granola (page 267) or Galaxy Granola with 1 piece seasonal fruit

Tea or coffee

OG option: If you haven't time to boil eggs in the morning, make yourself a quick smoothie with 2 scoops of hemp protein powder, 8 ounces rice milk, banana, and/or frozen or fresh berries.

MIDMORNING SNACK:

8-ounce glass kefir (soy kefir is fine)

LUNCH:

Lentil Salad (pages 276–278)

OG option: You can pick an easier salad from one of the other days or make this incredibly nutritious lentil salad ahead of time. It keeps well for 3 or 4 days.

MIDAFTERNOON SNACK:

1 Crispy Coconut and Flax Protein Bar (page 176)

Hot or iced green tea

DINNER:

Garlicky Mushrooms on Toast (page 317)

Baked apples with a dollop of plain yogurt

Mint tea with honey

WEEK TWO

Day One:

BEFORE BREAKFAST:

8-ounce glass lemon water (add the juice of 1/2 lemon to filtered water)

BREAKFAST:

Coconut Protein Pancakes (page 268)

If you haven't time to cook these pancakes in the morning, you may want to
swap with a weekend breakfast. You can also make the batter the night
before to make it superquick.

Tea or coffee

MIDMORNING SNACK:

Mango Smoothie: Peel and cube 1 mango. Place in blender with 4 ounces
almond or rice milk and 1/2 cup crushed ice. Blend until smooth.

LUNCH:

Crunchy Watercress Delight Salad (page 271)

Eat with a warm sprouted-grain tortilla

MIDAFTERNOON SNACK:

1 GG-recommended treat (page 57)

Iced or hot green tea

DINNER:

Quinoa Gado-Gado (page 296)

1 ounce of dark chocolate

Day Two:

BEFORE BREAKFAST:

8-ounce glass lemon water (add the juice of ½ lemon to filtered water)

BREAKFAST:

1 cup Nutty Granola (page 267) with homemade almond milk (page 267)
and ½ sliced banana

Tea or coffee

MIDMORNING SNACK:

Crispy Coconut and Flax Protein Bar (page 176)

OG option: Quick Protein Shake (page 63)

LUNCH:

Pasta salad: Boil some quinoa or whole-wheat spiral noodles, drain, and toss
with some extra virgin olive oil; add some chopped seasonal vegetables
(summer: tomatoes, bell peppers, and zucchini; winter: broccoli and
butternut squash). Add your dressing of choice.

OG tip: This salad is so quick and easy to make. I suggest making the pasta
the night before and adding the veggies before you go to work.

MIDAFTERNOON SNACK:

Handful of raw almonds and 4 or 5 dried apricots or figs

Iced or hot green tea

DINNER:

Vegetarian Chili (page 316)

Papaya or cantaloupe with a squeeze of lemon or lime

Day Three:

BEFORE BREAKFAST:

8-ounce glass lemon water (add the juice of ½ lemon to filtered water)

BREAKFAST:

Tempeh or eggs scrambled in olive oil with some chopped-up onion, bell peppers, and zucchini

OG option: ¾ cup of Kashi GoLean Cereal with almond milk and ½ sliced banana

MIDMORNING SNACK:

Gorgeously Green Smoothie (page 266)

LUNCH:

Large spinach salad with mushrooms, black olives, sprouts, radishes, cucumbers, ½ avocado, and 1 cut-up hard-boiled egg or baked tofu. Dress with GG Dressing (page 63).

MIDAFTERNOON SNACK:

1 slice sprouted-grain toast with a little almond butter

OG option: GG-recommended protein bar (page 45)

Iced or hot green tea

DINNER:

Teriyaki-glazed salmon or tempeh

I love this glaze because it works well for fish, tempeh, and tofu.

Combine ¼ cup tamari, 3 tbsp orange juice, 2 cloves minced garlic, 3 tbsp toasted sesame oil, 1 tbsp maple syrup, and salt and pepper to taste. Put the salmon or tempeh in the marinade and refrigerate for an hour or so. When ready to cook, heat some peanut oil in a skillet and sauté until cooked through, then add the leftover marinade and cook for an additional 3 minutes. Serve with steamed spinach or Swiss chard

1 cup applesauce with raisins and a spoonful of plain or soy yogurt

Mint tea

Day Four:

BEFORE BREAKFAST:

8-ounce glass lemon water (add the juice of ½ lemon to filtered water)

BREAKFAST:

1 cup steel-cut oatmeal, tsp shredded coconut, 1 tsp raw honey, and homemade almond milk (page 267)

Scatter some walnuts on top

MIDMORNING SNACK:

1 cut-up pear or apple and 6-ounce glass kefir

LUNCH:

Veggie Wrap: 1 sprouted-grain tortilla filled with lettuce, marinated bell
peppers, cucumber, and White Bean Hummus (page 291)

1 apple

MIDAFTERNOON SNACK:

Crispy Coconut and Flax Protein Bar (page 176)

Iced or hot green tea

DINNER:

Oven-Roasted Florentine Peppers (page 302)

Serve with 1 slice of crusty ciabatta or olive bread. Cut off 1 generous slice
per person and freeze the rest so you won't be tempted to eat more.
Splash out and buy the very best bread you can find because you won't
be eating very much bread on this diet—so best enjoy every morsel of
it while you can. The bread is a must for this recipe because it soaks up
the yummy juices after you've eaten the peppers. (If bell peppers aren't
in season, pick a dinner recipe for the appropriate season from Section
Eight.)

1 Miraculous Chocolate Macaroon (page 177) or 1 piece seasonal fruit

Mint tea

Day Five:

BEFORE BREAKFAST:

8-ounce glass lemon water (add the juice of ½ lemon to filtered water)

BREAKFAST:

1 Coconut, Walnut, and Banana Muffin (page 269) and ½ cup homemade
yogurt with 1 teaspoon honey

MIDMORNING SNACK:

8-ounce glass kefir

LUNCH:

Nutty Coleslaw (page 272) with a warm tortilla

MIDAFTERNOON SNACK:

1 apple with 1 tbsp almond butter
Iced or hot green tea

DINNER:

Kebabs with shrimp or chicken-style seitan (cut into chunks), bell peppers,
onions, and zucchini Thread onto a skewer and brush with olive oil.
Season with salt and pepper. Bake in a hot oven (400°F) for 30 minutes
or until brown. (If these vegetables aren't in season, pick a winter recipe
from Section Eight.)

1 cup cooked brown basmati rice. **Cook Once, Eat Twice.**

Mint tea

Day Six:

BEFORE BREAKFAST:

8-ounce glass lemon water (add the juice of ½ lemon to filtered water)

BREAKFAST:

2 slices sprouted-grain toast with almond butter and ½ sliced banana
½ cup plain or soy yogurt with honey

MIDMORNING SNACK:

Iced Café Latte (page 330)

LUNCH:

Waldorf Salad (page 270)

MIDAFTERNOON SNACK:

8 raw almonds and 3 dried prunes

Iced or hot green tea

DINNER:

Lentil and Cauliflower Stew (page 299)

1 ounce organic dark chocolate

Mint tea

Day Seven:

BEFORE BREAKFAST:

8-ounce glass lemon water (add the juice of ½ lemon to filtered water)

Water/aloe

BREAKFAST:

2 poached eggs

1 slice sprouted-grain toast

OG and Vegan option: 2 slices sprouted-grain toast with almond or apple
butter

Tea or coffee

MIDMORNING SNACK:

8-ounce smoothie with almond or rice milk, berries, 1 scoop hemp powder,
and 1 tsp honey

LUNCH:

Corn and Black Bean Salad (page 272)

MIDAFTERNOON SNACK:

Pick a Gorgeously Green treat (page 342) and enjoy!

DINNER:

Mushroom Risotto (page 316) with green salad

1 piece seasonal fruit

Mint tea

DEEP GREEN WEEK ONE SHOPPING LIST

Dairy/protein/dairy alternatives

1 box almond milk (or 1-pound bag raw almonds to make your own)

1 large container Lifeway or Rachel's Kefir (soy is fine)

1 dozen organic (omega-3) eggs

1 small package feta cheese

1 large container organic plain yogurt (or 1 gallon organic whole milk to make your own)

1 organic goat cheese log

1 large container hemp protein powder (Nutiva or Living Harvest)

1 medium container organic ricotta cheese

1 small carton buttermilk (O)

1 small packet organic butter/ soy spread for baking

1 small chunk raw Parmesan cheese

1 can Wild Planet low-mercury tuna (optional)

Produce

1 romaine lettuce (O)

1 head celery (O)

1 pound carrots (O)

1 cucumber (O)

1 package sprouts

1 bunch radishes (O)

Large portobello mushroom (1 per person)

1 bunch flat-leaf parsley

1 bunch fresh cilantro

1 bunch spinach (O)

3 yams (O)

7 lemons (O)

1 large head broccoli (O)

2 tomatoes (O)

1 bunch watercress

1 jicama

1 bag organic frozen berries

1 bunch organic bananas

1 mango

½ pound brown mushrooms

3 apples or pears

3 medium avocados

4 medium yellow onions

1 head Napa cabbage

2 parsnips

1 orange

1 small root fresh ginger (size of two fingers)

1 red bell pepper (if in season)

2 garlic bulbs

1 16-ounce bag green lentils

Oils/vinegars/nuts/seeds

1 32-fluid-ounce large bottle extra-virgin olive oil (organic and cold-pressed)

1 14-ounce jar virgin coconut oil

1 32-ounce bottle peanut oil

1 8-ounce bottle organic flaxseed oil

1 bottle organic apple cider vinegar

1 16-ounce bag raw almonds

1 16-ounce bag raw walnuts

1 16-ounce slivered almonds

1 jar organic almond butter

1 16-ounce bag pine nuts

Cereals/grains/pasta/rice

1 bag Galaxy Granola or Nutty Granola (page 267)

1 loaf sprouted-grain bread

1 box crackers (Doctor Kracker or Mary's Gone Crackers)

2 boxes quinoa pasta (penne or fusilli)

1 package sprouted-grain tortillas

1 bag organic basmati rice

1 bag organic short-grain brown rice (www.lundberg.com)

1 container steel-cut oatmeal

1 large carton organic rolled oats

1 box whole-wheat couscous

1 bag coconut flour (www.tropicaltraditions.com)

1 bag puffed brown rice

Extras

1 large bag shredded raw unsweetened coconut

1 jar raw honey

Tea and coffee, organic and fair-trade

Mint teabags, organic

1 jar black Kalamata olives

1 jar Dijon mustard

1 bar organic dark chocolate

1 small tin unsweetened cocoa powder

1 jar brown rice syrup

1 jar unsulphured molasses

1 bag dried apricots

1 bag dried cranberries

1 bag dried prunes

1 small bag raisins

2 cans black beans (www.eden.com)

4 cans garbanzo beans (www.eden.com) or 1 large bag of dried garbanzo beans

2 cans coconut milk

2 28-ounce cans tomatoes

1 glass jar organic applesauce

1 jar capers

1 jar sun-dried tomatoes

1 jar organic tahini

1 small box vegetable bouillon cubes or 3 boxes organic vegetable broth

1 bottle organic white cooking wine

DEEP GREEN WEEK TWO SHOPPING LIST

Dairy/dairy alternatives/protein
1 tub organic Greek yogurt
1 jar Spectrum mayonnaise
1 large container kefir
1 package WestSoy "Chicken Style" Seitan or 16 shrimp
1 package tempeh or 4 ounces wild Alaskan salmon (per person)
1 jar ghee or 4 sticks organic butter to make your own

Produce
4 apples (O)
2 Granny Smith apples
1 avocado
2 large bunches spinach (O)
1 papaya or cantaloupe melon (O)
1 large bag mushrooms
1 orange (O)
1 red bell pepper per person (if in season) (O)
2 medium zucchini (O)
1 large tomato (O)
6 scallions (O)
1 small red cabbage (O)
1 red onion
1 ear fresh corn or 1 bag frozen corn (O)
1 small head cauliflower
3 medium potatoes

Oils/vinegars/nuts/seeds
1 bottle rice vinegar (Asian section of store)
1 bottle toasted sesame oil
1 package sesame seeds

Cereals/pasta/grains/rice
1 loaf sprouted-grain bread
1 box quinoa
1 box arborio rice

Extras
1 16-ounces can Great Northern white beans
1 jar marinated red bell peppers
1 jar apple butter
1 bottle agave syrup
1 jar organic peanut butter
1 package dried mushrooms (available in most grocery stores)

Section Three
Gorgeously Lean and Green Meals

CHAPTER SEVEN

Dream Meal

It's a fantasy meal. I invite you to choose six people to have at your table (dead or alive and not family), and then you get to pick an appetizer, an entrée, and a dessert. The sky's the limit for what you can eat. Think of the best meal you have ever had in your life and go from there. Close your eyes and let your imagination soar. Go on; write it down—your dream meal.

My dream meal guests:
Shakespeare
Jesus
Maya Angelou
Julia Roberts
Oprah Winfrey
Vandana Shiva (eco-activist)

I know I've got the usual suspects on my list—Jesus and Shakespeare—but I really would love to pick their brains. Julia Roberts is a must—with her wicked sense of humor and deeply inquiring mind, she'll keep us all on our toes. I chose the author Maya Angelou because I love her and I think she would get on well with Shakespeare and have a great time with Vandana, and I chose Oprah because she would ask Jesus the best-ever questions, and she and Julia always have a blast.

So that's my group, and we're all going to sit under a heavenly pagoda, somewhere tropical, with fragrant jasmine blossoms hanging above our heads. And I'll plan a meal fit for the gods.

REDIRECT YOUR FOCUS

Rather than focusing on what you can't eat or what you don't like, I invite you to think about the foods you love as much as you want to. If you love butter croissants, as I do, think about them, salivate over them, because you are going to be able to eat one on this diet. Same goes for chocolate and whipped cream. Try to change the way you think about food, and don't ever feel bad when you catch yourself thinking about the tastes and textures that give you pleasure. It's natural and wonderful. So many women tell me that they love all the "wrong foods" or that they only have to *look* at a cookie to gain a few pounds. I think these girls are giving themselves a hard time, and I bet if they were to make a list of the foods they *really* love, they'd be surprised. A diet is a way of life, and the only way it's going to work forever is if you actually enjoy what you eat every day. I love cooking for friends. It gives me an excuse to push the boundaries and try new recipes or dishes I would never cook for a regular family meal. I've also learned that the less perfect my dinners are, the better. My friends loved my flourless chocolate cake that completely caved in because I took it out too early—it gave us an excuse to fill the giant crater with whipped cream. I've often forgotten vital ingredients or had to improvise at the last minute because I didn't read the recipe properly. These kinds of mistakes make for great stories, and everyone feels at home because, once in a while, we all mess up.

Now it's your chance to create something extraordinary. If you feel that your life lacks creativity, the best way to turn it around is to get into the kitchen. You get to be an alchemist in your own home—turning basic, raw ingredients into exquisite dishes.

This is your dream meal, and you get to prepare, cook, and serve it to some of your closest friends. The sky's the limit. The only rule is that you are the chef.

1. Dream in Green

Your dinner should be as Gorgeously Green as you can make it. Take everything you've discovered in the pages of this book and put it to good use.

Try to include as many eco-friendly aspects to this meal as you can:

- Include all the organic ingredients that you can possibly find. You may even want to look at purchasing organic wines, tea and coffee, and chocolate.

- Cook for the season: Make absolutely sure that the recipes you pick include ingredients that are ripe and perfect for the season. I avoid the summer vegetables red bell peppers and fresh tomatoes in the winter and go for squash, parsnips, and mushrooms instead.
- Create a meal with as many locally produced items as you can. It can be a lot of fun to make a project out of this. You should be able to find most of your meat and produce locally. However, items such as flour, dairy, and, obviously, spices will prove more of a challenge. At least go organic.

2. Plan the Event

What's the occasion? Does someone you love have a birthday coming up? Perhaps one of your friends has something else to celebrate: a new baby, a new job, a new house, or a promotion? Maybe one of your friends just needs cheering up with the most amazing surprise dinner she or he has ever tasted. So start thinking about the event. It may be that you just want to celebrate great food and invite four or five of your closest girlfriends.

If you're a bit nervous because you're not used to cooking for people, keep it simple and just invite one friend, or cook a romantic dinner for the love of your life. The only rule is that this be a delicious indulgence for everyone involved.

Having given it a bit of thought, consulted your calendar, and made a few phone calls, write down the event in the box below.

THE EVENT

- WHAT ARE YOU CELEBRATING?
- WHO IS INVITED?
- WHAT IS THE DATE?

3. Plan the Menu

This is the part that I love! The first thing to consider is the time of year because you don't want to be serving hot soups or heavy meat dishes in the summer, or gazpacho in winter. Because your first consideration is local and seasonal, you may want to take a trip to a farmer's market to see what's available. If you decide to serve a special meat or fish, you may need to find out if you must order it ahead of time.

Sample Menus:

In the box below, you will see the sample menus for your shade.

MY MENU

Three-Mushroom Fettucine
Wild Alaskan Salmon with an Herb Crust and Hollandaise Sauce
Peaches Rosebud
Miraculous Chocolate Macaroons

LIGHT GREEN MENU

Summer
Roasted Tomato Summer Soup with Basil Pesto
Angel Hair Pasta with Scallops
Pavlova

Winter
Creamy Carrot and Parsnip Soup
Citrus Roast Chicken
Steamed Chocolate Sponge

BRIGHT GREEN MENU

Summer
Arugula and Radicchio Salad
Herb-Crusted Salmon
Little Chocolate Pots

Winter
Waldorf Salad
Beef Stew
Baked Apples with Mascarpone Cream

DEEP GREEN MENU

Summer
Garlicky Cucumber Soup
Tolley's Summer Zucchini Pie
Flourless Chocolate Cake with Vanilla Soy Ice Cream

Winter
Black Bean Soup
Three-Mushroom Fettucine
Pomegranate, Banana, and Ginger Brûlée

4. The Invitation

Having decided on the event and the menu, it's time to send an invite. Even if it's a totally informal lunch for a girlfriend or a dinner for your partner, send a pretty invitation on recycled paper. The Green Field Paper Company makes the most beautiful seed-embedded recycled cards (www.greenfieldpaper.com), or send an invitation as an e-mail. A few months ago, I wanted to thank some neighborhood moms for helping me out with Lola while I was writing this book. I planned a light summer lunch and sent out an e-mail invitation to them. I spent hours preparing and making sure that every detail was attended to—from fun recycled paper place cards to scrumptious fair-trade chocolates as favors.

The meal was extremely inexpensive, for I used almost only seasonal vegetables: I prepared roasted tomato soup with pesto drizzle as an appetizer, leek and goat cheese tart as the entrée, and a fruit salad for dessert. It worked out to be just four dollars per head. It helped that I grow my own herbs, including basil for the pesto, and I make my own sparkling water with my soda stream machine (www.sodaclub usa.com). The biggest expense was the delicious organic white wine. We had a blast, and all agreed that a homemade ladies' lunch is a forgotten pleasure that we should enjoy more often.

CHAPTER EIGHT

Eating Out

It's all very well following an eating plan when you are at home, but what about those numerous occasions when you are on the road or eating out with friends? This is the real challenge: to maintain your new way of eating and carry it into every situation. Let the following guide help you.

FLYING

I travel quite a lot, and the biggest challenge is keeping my diet healthy when I'm in and out of airports and sitting in a cramped airplane with unhealthy snacks. It's all about preparation—especially since airlines don't provide food anymore, you're stuck with the prepackaged, limited choices that are available at airports.

- Say no to all the little free snacks (pretzels, nuts, chips, etc.) and the ones you pay for. They are covered in salt, which is the worst thing you can eat while flying because it will dehydrate you.
- Drink only water because soda will dehydrate you, and fruit juices are jam-packed with sugar. You need to drink 8 ounces of water for every hour in the air.
- Avoid alcohol at all costs. It will dehydrate you and make you feel terrible.
- Bring a mini–lunch box. (I found the smallest kid's insulated box imaginable—it's perfect.) Pack it with a sandwich and mini–plastic

containers of raw nuts, healthy crackers, and fruit. Whenever I unpack
my lunch box, I always get envious glances from fellow passengers who
are faced with either an expensive dry-looking roll or nothing.

- Bring a reusable travel mug. The air attendant will rinse it out and refill
  it for you.

ON THE ROAD

If you have a long commute or take a lot of road trips, again, it's all about preparation. You don't want to find yourself hungry and then stopping at a gas station to
buy something that you'll regret eating. Remember, thinking ahead and bringing
your own will save your money and your health. Avoid drive-through restaurants
at all costs—it's a high price to pay for packaging, your pocketbook, and your
health.

- Keep a can or bag of raw almonds and a couple of protein energy bars in
  your glove compartment. You never know when you may need them.
- Make sandwiches that are easy to eat. You don't want a glob of tuna
  mayo landing on your lap. Thinly sliced turkey or almond butter and
  jelly are good choices.
- A crunchy organic apple is great for a car ride, or bags of carrots and
  peanut butter–filled celery sticks.
- Always take a reusable coffee mug so you can get refills on the road.
- Take a large reusable water bottle (www.camelbak.com).

IN AN EMERGENCY

There are times when we get stuck somewhere and have to content ourselves with
whatever food is available. I have found myself stranded at many an airport, have
been stuck for hours on a freeway moving five miles per hour or sitting at a tediously
long soccer game. In these situations, I am so grateful to find my secret "emergency"
stash in the recesses of my purse. I almost always carry a couple of protein bars or
dried fruit nut bars (www.larabar.com) and a small bag of raw almonds.

CAUGHT SHORT

If you find yourself without a secret stash or a homemade snack, especially on an airport layover, I suggest that you:

- Pick the vegetarian option at a deli because they rarely use high-quality, nitrate-free meats or low-mercury tuna.
- Try to avoid too much packaging. Have them wrap your sandwich in paper, and avoid the bag and any condiments, plastic flatware, and napkins that you won't use.

RESTAURANTS

I love eating out and occasionally getting a respite from doing the dishes. However, I've started saving a great deal of money by cooking at home at least half the time. The beauty of this is that I now really look forward to eating out; before, it was just something we did all the time.

I try to pick the healthiest restaurants in the area and always Google "healthy/organic restaurants" before visiting a new city. I often call ahead and ask how much of their food is locally sourced and organic. If I'm going to spend my hard-earned cash on a restaurant, I want to make sure it's worth it.

Lessen your eco-impact by saying "no, thanks" to water, unless you are really thirsty. Restaurants and diners often give you a glass of tap water, regardless of whether you want it or not, and then they keep filling it up—that's a lot of water that's just thrown down the drain.

RESTAURANT—BUFFET

I try to avoid buffets because they always encourage me to overeat. I also don't trust how long the food has been sitting out. I have had very bad food poisoning twice from a salad buffet. Buffets also involve a lot of waste because, after the second or third helping, I tend to just pick. It's typical to see a lot of barely touched plates left at the table after a buffet. As our eyes can be bigger than our stomachs, all that good food is scraped off into large trash cans and taken straight to the landfill. If you find yourself at a buffet:

- Don't attempt to pile up an enormous plate of everything you can get your hands on. It's a buffet, so you can cherry-pick, going back a forth a few times to get tiny portions of whatever you fancy. Use a salad plate instead of an entrée plate to encourage these smaller portions.
- Start with a salad dressed with olive oil and vinegar; then wait a few minutes before your next course.
- Slow down—buffet eaters often get into a total frenzy! Give yourself at least five minutes between courses.
- Avoid bread and crackers, and fill up on fresh fish and veggies instead.

AMERICAN RESTAURANT

If you find yourself at a restaurant where the food source is not specified (i.e., grass-fed beef from Oregon or wild Alaskan salmon), you can be sure the meat will *not* be grass-fed or organic and the salmon *will* be farmed. The best meat choice would be lamb, because it contains the least amount of hormones and antibiotics and is very often grass-fed.

- Pick lamb or duck if the restaurant does not specify that its meat is organic. Second choice would be fish, and third choice, chicken. I never eat beef at a restaurant unless I absolutely know that it's organic.
- Ask if any of their food is sourced locally and/or is organic.
- If they don't have a vegetarian dish that takes your fancy, ask for a vegetable plate, which is often delicious.
- Choose a salad made with romaine lettuce (Caesar salad) rather than a salad made with iceberg lettuce. The nutritional content of romaine is five times higher than that of iceberg.
- Avoid the bread basket unless it's the most incredible artisan and locally baked bread. In that case, you may want to treat yourself to one slice or a roll before asking them to remove the basket!
- Pick out vegetables that are in season.
- Choose only fish that is sustainable (good idea to always keep your seafood-watch pocket guide in your wallet [www.seafoodwatch.org]). Best choices depend on your region. However, the following choices will lessen your eco-impact:

- Catfish (U.S.-farmed)
- Clams, mussels, oysters (farmed)
- Halibut (Pacific)
- Wild salmon (Alaskan)
- Tilapia (U.S.-farmed)
- Scallops: bay (U.S.-farmed)
- Lobster: spiny (U.S.)
- Pollock (wild Alaskan)
- Trout: rainbow (farmed)
- Eat only half of what you are served and ask that the remainder be boxed up to take home. Beware, though, of polystyrene boxes (ask first) because chemicals can migrate into hot or warm food.

CHINESE

- First question is: Do they use MSG? They may well tell you they don't when the truth is that they often slip it in for flavor, so if you are sensitive or allergic to food additives, it's best to avoid Chinese takeout food.
- Pick vegetable-, soy-, and tofu-based dishes rather than meat. You can be almost sure that their meat will not be good quality.
- Ask for brown rice instead of white.
- If you're getting food to go, say no to any utensils and minipackets of soy sauce that you know you won't use.
- Pick a restaurant that doesn't use polystyrene containers so you can avoid any chemicals leaching into your hot food. Also keep in mind that polystyrene doesn't decompose.
- Remember to recycle any clean paper packaging.

JAPANESE

Most everyone I know loves sushi, but we need to be savvy about its eco-impact.

- Be extremely careful about avoiding mercury-laden fish. It's a good idea to visit www.nrdc.org/health/effects/mercury/index.asp and calculate exactly how much of your favorite fish you can safely eat. As a general rule, avoid all kinds of tuna when eating out.

- Try to choose only sustainable fish.
- Drink a huge bowl of miso soup to start—it's healthy and filling.

Best Sushi Choices for Lessening Your Eco-Impact

EAT AS MUCH AS YOU WANT	EAT OCCASIONALLY	AVOID
Amaebi (spot prawns—Canada)	Flounder/sole (Pacific)	Ebi (imported shrimp and prawns)
Suzuki (farmed striped bass)	Sea scallops (U.S./Canada) Ika (squid)	Hamachi (farmed yellow-tail—Australia/Japan)
Uni (sea urchin—Canada)	Kani (king crab)	Hirame (flounder/sole—Atlantic)
Surimi (Alaska pollock—U.S.)	Kanikama (imitation crab)	Hon maguro (bluefin tuna)
Sake (wild Alaskan salmon)	Tai (red porgy—U.S.)	Ikura (roe from Atlantic farmed salmon)
Ikura (wild Alaskan salmon roe)	Uni (sea urchin from California)	Maguro (bigeye/yellowfin tuna)
Masago (capelin smelt roe—Iceland)		Sake (Atlantic-farmed salmon)
		Tako (octopus)
		Toro (bluefin tuna and yellowfin tuna—imported longline)
		Unagi (freshwater eels)

MEXICAN

- Avoid ordering meat; it's unlikely to be good quality.
- Order rice, beans, veggies, and salad.
- If weight loss is an issue, avoid the tortilla chips and margaritas. They both have a high caloric content.

- Enjoy the guacamole—it'll make your skin glow.
- Go easy on the cheese because it's unlikely to be good quality.

ITALIAN/GREEK

- If you feel like meat, order lamb. It's often on the menu of Italian restaurants.
- When ordering grilled meat or fish, ask that it be grilled with little or no butter or oil
- If you're ordering pasta, ask for one-half of a portion or an appetizer-size portion. U.S. portions are way too large.
- Keep away from the bread basket, especially if you are eating pasta.
- If weight loss is an issue, stay away from creamy sauces because they'll already have put a bunch of butter or oil in the dish to make it taste good.
- Order only fresh tomato dishes if it's summer. Out-of-season tomatoes carry a heavy eco-impact and don't taste great.
- In a Greek restaurant, order slices of cucumber rather than pita bread to mop up the hummus and eggplant dip.
- Order soup as an appetizer.
- Order fresh fruit sorbet instead of gelato as a dessert.

INDIAN

- It's easy to be vegetarian in an Indian restaurant: Go crazy picking all the yummy veggie dishes, especially lentil dahl.
- If weight loss is an issue, go easy on the naan bread and papadums. Also avoid the deep-fried appetizers like samosas and onion bhajees.
- If you really want meat, pick lamb. It's less likely to be laced with hormones and antibiotics.
- Raita, which is a yogurt side dish, is prepared with cucumber and sometimes mint and is a great accompaniment to almost every Indian dish. It's low in fat, delicious, and cools down the hot spices in the curry and tandoori dishes.

DELI/SANDWICH BAR

- Try to go veggie, for meats will likely contain nitrates in almost all delis.
- Avoid tuna, because it's sure not to be low in mercury.
- Go easy on the mayo. Have it spread lightly on one slice of the sandwich only.
- Include mustard, olive tapenade, pesto, sun-dried tomatoes, and pickles to give your sandwich or salad flavor.
- Pick egg or egg salad for your protein source.
- Avoid chips, even if they say "fat-free" or "zero trans fats."
- Avoid individually packaged sandwiches, crackers, or cookies.
- Take only the flatware, napkins, and condiments that you know you will use.
- If you know you are going to the deli, take along a plastic reusable container for your salad, sandwich, or cold cuts.

CHAPTER NINE

Pantry Purge

One of the things that propelled me into healthy eating was the fact that I wanted to *feel* better. I realized that eating processed foods containing sugar and additives made me feel irritable, sluggish, agitated, or just plain awful in my own skin. A bit of takeout junk food assuaged my taste buds for about five minutes, but then I had to deal with how I felt half an hour later—not good *at all*. I had circles under my eyes, I didn't want to exercise, and I felt a bit depressed.

Bad food can be a downward spiral that can put us in a bleak place. In many studies, it has even been linked to serious depression. Some of the psychological studies of nutrition are fascinating: Two or three large ones have been done on prison inmates. One such study was conducted by a professor of criminal justice, Dr. Stephen Schoenthaler. He researched 8,000 teenagers in nine different correctional facilities that replaced a diet high in sugar and refined carbohydrates with one high in fruits, veggies, and whole grains. During the year, violent and antisocial incidents decreased by almost half.

This kind of study shows us that even if our bad moods don't land us in prison, they can do much to ruin a precious day, and that there's not a better mood enhancer than good nutrition and exercise. Further, we can be seriously affected by some of the additives, preservatives, and dyes in processed and convenience food. The Feingold Program (www.feingold.org) has made an in-depth study of how many food additives adversely affect our health. They address a myriad of health concerns—from behavioral problems in children to serious allergies and skin problems in adults. The program eschews the use of any artificial coloring, artificial flavoring, aspartame, and the artificial preservatives BHA, BHT, and TBHQ. It's interesting to visit their Web site and read some of the success stories and to see just how many foods these petroleum-based chemicals are hidden in. I'm currently working on getting a summer camp that which Lola attends to replace the contents of their snack and candy cupboard with healthier alternatives. I talked to Lola about it and, amazingly, she didn't think it was a bad idea—aside from the daylight robbery of using three dollars of her precious pocket money for a small candy bar, she also said that she might have a bit more energy for the requisite singing and dancing if she ate something healthier. Kids are *very* smart!

FOOD ADDITIVES

Without a cornucopia of additives, processed foods wouldn't look or taste the way they do: Cakes and marshmallows would be as hard as rock; meats and vegetables would be soft and gray; instant oatmeal wouldn't work the way its supposed to when you add the water. Actually, you wouldn't want to buy *anything* processed if it weren't for these chemicals, which give highly processed food the appearance of real food, and old food the appearance of fresh food. There would be nothing wrong with tasty-looking food if it weren't for the fact that many of these additives can be pretty bad for your health. As is true for skin care, the toxic effects of these chemicals won't kill you after one serving. But many of them accumulate in your fatty tissue, so if you eat them every day, you may be putting yourself at risk for a plethora of unpleasant conditions, including hypoglycemia, asthma, eczema, and depression.

I invite you to start becoming hyperaware of these additives, what they are, and what they do, so that you can make informed choices. Have a good look at the list below—these are the worst offenders and you'll be healthier and happier without them.

1. SODIUM NITRITE OR NITRATE

This is used as a preservative and also a taste and color enhancer in meat. It is typically found in bacon, sausage, hot dogs, luncheon meats, and canned meats.

Nitrates can form potentially carcinogenic nitrosamines in your body, and studies have shown that they can cause prostate, stomach, and breast cancer. Some food companies have been adding ascorbic acid to nitrate-treated meat to slow the formation of nitrates in the stomach. This has gone some way toward minimizing the harm that nitrates cause but hasn't eliminated it altogether. I always choose nitrate-free meat.

2. BHA AND BHT (BUTYLATED HYDROXYANISOLE AND BUTYLATED HYDROXYTOLUENE)

These chemicals are typically found in potato chips, vegetable oils, cereal, chewing gum, and soup bases. They are potentially harmful to the liver and kidneys and can cause allergic reactions. They can also cause neurological problems.

3. PROPYL GALLATE

This additive stops fats and oils from going rancid. It is often used with BHA and BHT and is typically found in processed meats, chicken stock/broth, and even chewing gum. It is a suspected carcinogen.

4. MSG (MONOSODIUM GLUTAMATE)

Most of you have heard of this flavor enhancer—I regularly get Chinese restaurant flyers in my mailbox that say "no MSG"—so people have obviously caught on. But be aware that even if it's not listed on the ingredients, it can come under the guise of "natural flavoring," "spices," or "seasoning." Read a label and sometimes you'll discover it in canned soups, salad dressings, spice and flavoring blends (in rice and noodle dishes), and hydrolyzed vegetable protein (HVP). It has been linked in studies to sudden cardiac arrest in athletes and, on a less dramatic level, often causes severe headaches and nausea. No wonder I used to feel awful after a Chinese takeout in my student days.

5. HYDROGENATED OR PARTIALLY HYDROGENATED VEGETABLE OILS

These oils have gotten a lot of bad press over the last few years, and there is good reason. They are a kind of saturated fat, which raises the bad cholesterol and can lead to heart disease. Also known as trans fats, these fats also lower the good cholesterol, which we need for the formation of cell membranes and hormones. Many studies also point to other serious health implications. The situation is so dire that the World Health Organization has tried to remove them in some parts of the world; they have been banned in three U.S. states. To find out more about trans fats and how to avoid them, visit www.bantransfat.com. These nasty fats are found in many foods—frozen meals, baked goods, cookies, crackers, doughnuts. Unless the label says "no trans fats," the food probably contains it.

6. ASPARTAME (NUTRASWEET AND EQUAL)

This ubiquitous sweetener is responsible for 75 percent of all FDA food-related complaints, which include headaches, nausea, memory loss, seizures, vision loss—even cancer. There have been many aspartame lawsuits that accuse companies using aspartame of poisoning. The suits allege that the accused food companies committed fraud and breach of warranty by marketing products to the public with full knowledge that aspartame, the sweetener, is a neurotoxin. These companies include manufacturers of diet sodas and sugar-free foods and candies.

7. ACESULFAME-K (SUNETT AND SWEET ONE)

This artificial sweetener is two hundred times sweeter than sugar. It is found in baked goods, soft drinks, and chewing gum. Two studies with rats found it to cause cancer. Further studies are needed to see if it affects humans in the same way—but I'm not taking the risk!

8. FOOD COLORINGS (BLUE 1 AND 2; RED 3; GREEN 3; YELLOW 6)

These dyes have been found to cause a plethora of health problems—from cancer to thyroid problems in animal studies. It only makes sense to avoid them. European tests have found these same dyes to cause serious behavioral problems in children.

9. OLESTRA

This is a synthetic fat that stops fat from being absorbed by the body. It also prevents essential vitamins from being absorbed. It is mainly found in potato chips, and there have already been more than 15,000 complaints filed with the FDA from people suffering all kinds of symptoms, including vomiting and diarrhea.

10. POTASSIUM BROMATE

This chemical is found in breads and pizza dough and is a known carcinogen. The FDA has urged bakers to stop using it. Many companies have started phasing it out, yet many companies still use it. Numerous grocery chains have switched to using bromate-free processes, but some still use potassium bromate, and many fast-food chains use it in their burger buns.

11. HIGH-FRUCTOSE CORN SYRUP

This is in everything imaginable—ketchup, relishes, cakes, crackers, and drinks. It's pretty hard to avoid. I went into an enormous grocery store and could find only one item from four aisles of crackers, cookies, and baked goods that didn't contain it. The one item was a box of Ry Krisp crackers. It is often attributed as the cause of obesity, and I think that has to be the case: As Michael Pollan says in his remarkable book *The Omnivore's Dilemma*, "Since 1985, an American's annual consumption of

HFCS has gone from forty-five pounds to sixty-six pounds. You might think that this growth would have been offset by a decline in sugar consumption, since HFCS often replaces sugar, but that didn't happen: During the same period our consumption of refined sugar actually went up by five pounds. What this means is that we're eating and drinking all that high-fructose corn syrup *on top of* the sugars we were already consuming. In fact, since 1985 our consumption of all added sugars—cane, beet, HFCS, glucose, honey, maple syrup, whatever—has climbed from 128 pounds per person to 158 pounds."

If you factor in the change of our lifestyle since the 1980s, we are a much more sedentary society. Where children used to be out playing sports, they are now glued to a computer or TV screen for four or five hours a day. It's no wonder that more than 60 percent of Americans now meet the criteria for being overweight or obese.

12. SODIUM CHLORIDE (TABLE SALT)

Not all salts are equal. Refined table salt has had all the beneficial minerals and trace elements stripped out of it. It's also likely to contain aluminum as a drying agent. Aluminum is a toxic metal considered by some researchers to be linked to Alzheimer's disease. Unfortunately, refined salt is commonly used in most prepared foods, including cheese, pickles, and soy sauce. Make sure that you buy sea salt for home use.

13. SULFITES

Potassium sulfite and sodium bisulfite reduce discoloration in foods such as dried fruit, dehydrated soup or noodle mixes, syrups, pickles, shrimp, cookies, crackers, and beet sugar. It is also found in red wine and beer. Some people can be sulfite sensitive, which may result in a number of symptoms, including an acute asthma attack, a headache, a cough, and a skin rash. I think it's best to stay away from foods containing sulfites whenever possible.

14. EVAPORATED CANE JUICE

Although this is not a chemical additive per se, it's worth mentioning that "evaporated cane juice" is added to more foods that I am happy with: breakfast cereals, cheese crackers, supposedly healthy cereal bars, and soups and sauces. It's a kind of raw sugar made from sugarcane juice. But other than a few trace minerals, it is no better for you than regular sugar, which is highly caloric and messes with your blood sugar, leading to your getting fat. So try to find foods without it—hard, I know!

PURGE

With these fourteen additives to avoid fresh in your mind, take yourself and your book to your pantry and begin reading labels. Go through everything, looking at all the ingredients on cereal and cracker boxes, cans of soup, boxes of rice—basically anything in a can, box, or bag—and note if they contain any of the above. If they do, put them out on your kitchen table, or the floor so that you have more space to work with. You have two choices: Either make up a box to take to your local food bank (your local church will have one) or use up what you can't afford to give up right now.

My first "pantry purge" was a complete education and long overdue. I found old boxes of cake mix from I don't know when, and fancy tins of cheese crackers that had come in a holiday basket half a decade ago. It taught me a lesson not only about waste but also about ingredient horrors. What started as an activity that my husband wasn't thrilled about (coming home and not being able to even *step* into the kitchen) became a fascinating endeavor for both of us—he started delighting in finding a hidden ingredient that I had missed in a jar of jelly or asking me questions about impossibly complicated dye numbers. All in all, we felt incredibly satisfied as we piled the "good" food back into freshly wiped-out cupboards, but we felt bad that the food pantry, as grateful as they would be, would have to suffice with boxes of additives.

FREEZER BURN

Plan to spend an hour or so going through your fridge and freezer. On my last freezer purge, I couldn't believe what I found tucked away in the dark recesses. I laid it all out on the kitchen floor and decided not to buy another thing until we had eaten absolutely everything. It taught me a lesson: not to buy anything for the freezer that is not on my plan. I often think I'm stocking up for emergencies or unexpected guests, but many of those items just end up getting pushed farther and farther back. I found a cherry tart, coconut shrimp (with horrible freezer burn), and a wad of unlabeled meat covered in an impenetrable layer of frost. Why on earth did I buy the coconut shrimp? I think it was because Lola had mentioned that she loved it. Oh, yes, there were also two bags of very old collard greens that I had bought in a fit of sympathy for my Southern husband but that I never mustered up the strength to cook—I'm not a huge fan of collards. Grits I can face, but he'll have to go home for the rest!

Plan a couple of meals around the floor's spread. Some of you may have very little, and if that's the case, make sure you are using up everything from your pantry. The goal for the purging exercise is to clean out your entire kitchen so that you can start anew. A purge is also a great wake-up call to how much waste we produce not just in food but also in packaging. It can be heartbreaking to have to throw away a freezer-burned steak, yet it is a good reminder to stick to a weekly eating plan and a shopping list from now on.

LETTING GO

It's funny that sometimes the hardest things to let go of are the very things that make us feel awful. A tub of sugary ice cream can still find its way onto my lap while I'm watching TV. And an entire bread basket in a restaurant can disappear over a heated conversation with a girlfriend. At least I can control what I bring into my home, and I have to be vigilant about keeping *only* the good stuff in my kitchen. If cookies, chips, ice cream, or sodas are hanging around, they tend to be the first to get eaten while the organic produce rots away in the crisper drawer.

There are very few rules, for this is not a diet that you should grin and bear until you can get back to your regular life. It's a lifestyle change that I hope will stay with you forever. There are, however, a few foods that I invite you to avoid if you want to feel fantastic. Every small bad habit you let go of is a huge gain for your health, and I will give you yummy alternatives.

YOUR HEALTH IS REFLECTED IN YOUR GROCERY CART

If you want to feel better, there are a number of foods that I recommend you avoid. The processing and packaging of these foods gives them a heavy eco-impact. They all contain additives and/or an amount of sugar that will make you feel awful or pack on unnecessary pounds. When you next go to the grocery store, sneak a peek into other people's carts. I have never seen a bright-eyed, slim woman with fantastic energy pushing a cart full of processed foods. Conversely, I have seen hundreds of sad and gray-looking men and women standing in line with their carts overflowing with chips, crackers, sodas, and frozen meals. Fresh, minimally processed food puts a spring in your step and a sparkle in your eye.

Fill Your Cart with These:

High-energy/low-eco-impact foods (that will make you smile)

Raw fruits—High in vitamins, enzymes, fiber, and complex carbs

Vegetables—High in vitamins, enzymes, phytonutrients, and fiber

Berries—High in antioxidants

Sprouts—High in phytonutrients

Avocados—Healthy oils

Whole grains—Vitamins, high in fiber and healthy oils

Sprouted grains—High in vitamins and fiber

Raw nuts—Healthy oils and antioxidants

Seeds (sesame, hemp, flax)—Healthy oils, vitamins, and high in fiber

Fish oils (sardines, wild salmon)—Healthy oils for your heart and brain

Beans (kidney, pinto, black, and navy beans)—High in protein, fiber, and vitamins

Organic dairy—High in protein, vitamins, and enzymes

Avoid at All Costs:

Low-energy/high-eco-impact foods (that will make you sad)

Processed meats—High in sodium, nitrates, MSG, and other preservatives

Sodas—Chemical sweeteners that can adversely affect your health

Doughnuts and pastries—Hydrogenated oils, refined flour, no fiber

Canned soups—MSG, high in sodium and other preservatives

Flavored snacks and chips—MSG, high-fructose corn syrup, and artificial colors

Salad dressings—Added sugars, MSG

Diet and meal shakes—Added sugar and preservatives

Shortening and margarine—Hydrogenated oils

Instant rice and grains—Lack fiber and use refined grains

Breakfast cereals—High in sugar

Cookies and crackers—High in sugar and hydrogenated oils

ECO-IMPACT OF SUGAR

One of the unique ecosystems in the United States is Florida's Everglades, but the delicate ecology is being seriously compromised after decades of sugarcane farming. Tens of thousands of acres of the Everglades have been converted from subtropical forest to lifeless marshland, owing to excessive fertilizer runoff and irrigation drainage.

Juice pouches and boxes—High-fructose corn syrup and artificial colors

Frozen fried foods—MSG and hydrogenated oils

Also Avoid:

Sugary ice-blended drinks from the coffee shop (very expensive and fattening)

Sugary (sherbet added) smoothies from juice bars (very expensive and fattening)

Pre-prepared meals from grocery stores, including frozen meals (You're paying for the packaging and marketing rather than the food.)

Fast foods (from all fast-food chains—you know the culprits!)

Individually packaged items (such as kids' lunch box items), because they involve an enormous amount of packaging, which is not good for your eco-impact, and are more expensive

FRESH, FROZEN, OR CANNED VEGETABLES

FRESH—It's always best to buy fresh vegetables whenever you can because they contain more nutrients. However, if they look old or wilted, you may be better off with frozen veggies.

FROZEN—Read the ingredients on frozen packages to make sure that no salt was added. The vegetables are frozen when very fresh, so you're better off buying from the freezer aisle when certain fresh vegetables are out of season. Good choices include green beans, corn, peas, edamame, berries, and sliced bell peppers.

CANNED—This is my last choice because the high temperatures needed for the canning process can affect heat-sensitive and water-soluble nutrients. Sodium may also be added. Be mindful as well that most canning facilities use cans with a lining that can leach the hormone-disrupting chemical BPA into the food. Eden Foods (www.edenfoods.com) is an exception.

Finally, except for beans, canned fruits and vegetables are soggy and gray compared to their fresh and frozen counterparts.

CHAPTER TEN

Scouting It Out

Having established what to avoid and what to look for, it's time to investigate what's available in your area. I am well aware that many of you may not have access to a great selection of organic and sustainable foods, so we need to find a way of making this work for everybody.

Over the next week, go to your local grocery store, take a pad of paper and a pen, and find out what exactly is available.

USEFUL EXERCISE

Either take your book with you to the store or download the shopping list for your eating plan at www.gorgeouslygreen.com/shopping. With the lists in hand, visit your nearest stores and see if they carry the items you are going to need. It's worth taking the time to do this exercise because you can start comparing prices. I was looking for organic heavy cream and found a huge price discrepancy between the two stores that carry it in my area. I keep a price comparison spiral pad. It's small enough to fit in my purse, and every time I'm at the store, I whip it out to write down the latest prices of items that I regularly buy.

I have four main grocery stores within a five-mile radius of where I live and, annoyingly, they all have different strengths: One has a pretty good but expensive selection of organic produce, one carries reasonably priced organic milk, and I have to go to the farthest one to get organic meat and decent fish. Because I can't get it all in one place, I have to be really organized on a weekly basis.

SCORECARD

I highly recommend that you see how all the places where you can buy food in your area compare to one another in a number of different aspects. Fill in the scorecard on page 142 and see which place scores highest. Simply give each store a score from 1 to 5 (5 being the highest) on how they rate in these five areas: quality, organic selection, local/seasonal selection, cost, convenience.

Check out my scorecard below.

	TRADER JOE'S	RALPH'S	WHOLE FOODS	SMART & FINAL	FARMER'S MARKET
Quality	4	2	4	2	5
Organic Selection	2	2	5	1	4
Local/ Seasonal Selection	2	0	5	0	5
Cost	3	2	1	5	3
Convenience	4	3	3	3	2
Score	15	9	18	11	19

Now it's your turn to fill in your scores—as you can see from my example, it was a pretty close call. The farmer's market won out, which tells me that I should plan to do as much of my shopping there as possible.

	STORE 1	STORE 2	STORE 3	STORE 4	STORE 5
Quality					
Organic Selection					
Local/ Seasonal Selection					
Cost					
Convenience					
Score					

LIGHT GREEN SCOUT

Label reading for additives and the organic thing may be new to you. Most women are good at reading labels for calories, fats, and sugar content, but I want you to try to ignore these calculations in favor of focusing on the *quality* of a given food. Just trust that if it's a fresh, organic whole food, you'll be able to eat it on this diet. Go to your local store and make a list of every organic item you can find that is something you would enjoy. If there isn't anything organic, ask to speak to the manager and ask whether he or she is considering carrying some organic items in the future, and tell the manager what items you would like to see. (Take your book and read from the list of the most important foods to buy organic on page 245.)

Go to the cookie, cracker, and bread aisle and see if you can find some items that *don't* contain HFCS (high-fructose corn syrup) and other additives from the list starting on page 132. If you find anything that fits within the parameters of this diet, write it down. Finally, see if any stores around you carry organic and grass-fed meat or poultry.

BRIGHT GREEN SCOUT

You may already know if your local stores carry organic food, but take it a little further. Take your pad of paper and write down the organic items that they actually carry. Take notice if they carry mainly seasonal produce, and read labels to see whether or not anything is produced locally (you may have to ask the manager).

Pick up every item that you normally throw in your cart, and read every single ingredient—if it contains any of the additives mentioned on pages 132–135, write it down, and put a line through it to remind yourself that you won't be buying that item anymore. I recently found a brand of juice that a lot of Lola's friends have at school. I read every ingredient and couldn't believe how many additives were included. Be prepared for some surprises.

DEEP GREEN SCOUT

I would imagine that you often shop in health food stores. However, you may want to check out your regular grocery stores this week to see which organic products they are now offering—you may find a bargain or two.

Take your eco-friendliness a step further this week by committing to buy as much locally produced and fair-trade food as you can. If you are vegetarian or vegan, you may find it really tough to eat only locally produced food, as your diet will need protein from a variety of sources. Where does your tempeh or seitan come from? Is it genetically modified? If it doesn't say, how can you find out? How many additives can you find in your soy-based products?

Your job is to start asking a lot of questions!

AVAILABILITY

Having done your research, you are now faced with the stark facts about what is available and, more to the point, what is *not*. Now is a good time to go beyond the grocery store and find out what is available at farmer's markets, coops, or CSAs (community supported agriculture) in your area. Fortunately, the Internet has made this very easy for you. Simply log on to www.localharvest.org and you will find everything you need. I love this Web site because you simply type in your zip code and then choose either "farm" or "CSA," and all your nearest sources will come up. I confess, I spend way too long on the Web site because I'm thrilled by all the incredible farms that are relatively nearby. I want to visit them all and take Lola with me to get a taste of where and how our food is really produced.

First look up CSAs, because these communities offer a weekly or a monthly box of whatever they have. Either they will deliver it to your door or arrange a drop-off point, where you can go and pick it up. You are basically buying a share in the farm at a set price, with payment due ahead of time or on a seasonal basis. This Web site will tell you exactly how much your share will cost. Most offer the option of buying in for a year or six months. At first glance, it seems pricey, but trust me, if you were to add up these items on your grocery receipt, they would probably come to more. If you like to be surprised, the produce boxes are fun, for you never know what you'll get. I prefer to know ahead of time, because I need to plan the week's meals. I love subscribing to the meat and poultry farms because I know what I'll be getting and exactly when—this way I can plan my menus around this incredible meat, which will arrive just when I expect it.

Look up farms next because you may be surprised that there is a family farm within reasonable driving distance. Although they may not deliver, it could make for a fun trip for your family, and if they have a bunch of great stuff in season, you can buy a truckload and freeze it. A trip to a farm is also really informative and will inspire you to become even more food conscious.

The great thing about this Web site is that you'll see a map with dots all over it, delineating where the CSAs, farms, shops, and restaurants are, all over the country, and it's heartening to see that there are thousands and thousands of them dotted throughout the states.

Another fantastic Web site, this one for finding great pasture-raised meat, is www.eatwild.com. You'll be able to find loads of really great information here, too.

UPGRADING YOUR STAPLES

Now you are ready to restock your freezer, fridge, and pantry. Your eating-plan shopping lists should act as a great guide for what to get. Although I advise sticking to these shopping lists to avoid waste, the following items are a excellent idea in case you get stuck. You should be able to rustle up a delicious meal from these all-weather staples:

Pantry

Canned fish: Low-mercury tuna (Wild Planet or American Tuna), sardines, wild Alaskan salmon, and anchovies
Canned organic tomatoes
Canned organic tomato paste
Bottle of good-quality extra-virgin olive oil

Bottle of pure olive oil

Bottle of grape seed or expeller-pressed canola oil

Jar of virgin coconut oil

Small bottle of balsamic vinegar

Jar of organic sun-dried tomatoes

Jar of marinated bell peppers

Jar of pitted Kalamata olives

Jar of capers

Cans of organic garbanzo beans

Cans of organic black beans

Cans of coconut milk

Vegetable and chicken bouillon cubes

Organic whole-wheat pasta

Organic brown rice

Jar of honey

Jar of organic almond butter

Jar of tahini

Bag of raw almonds or walnuts

Bags of dried fruit

Box of vegetable bouillon cubes

Freezer

Bags of frozen organic mixed berries

Bags of frozen organic peas and green beans

Bag of organic edamame

Whole-wheat flour (should be kept in freezer to stop it from going rancid)

CHAPTER ELEVEN

Saving Money

LEAN AND GREEN

The Gorgeously Green Diet is not cost prohibitive. On the contrary, it is specifically designed with a tight budget in mind. I've taken a leaf out of my mom's book and become quite the thrifty girl. Mom was always frugal, not in a scrooge sense but in a thoughtful sense. It's now called being green, but back then it was just plain common sense. Nothing was wasted in the kitchen, for every item of food was considered valuable. If you've ever been rationed, as my parents were as children, you just can't throw food away.

In the United States we are used to relatively cheap food from massive industrial processors churning out heavily processed calories. This food is, however, expensive in the long run because we the consumers have to pay the price of having dirty air, soil, and water, and subsequently, ill health. We spend a smaller proportion of our income on our food than virtually any other non-third-world nation, and we pay the highest health care costs. Good-quality "real" food is preventive health care at it's best.

When food prices are high, we tend to eat more fattening foods, because low-quality crackers, cakes, and cookies are seemingly the least-expensive items on the shelf. However, this doesn't have to be the case. Bags of dried beans, rice, and fresh veggies like cabbages and beautiful root vegetables are bursting with the nutrition we need for wellness and can always be found at rock-bottom prices.

You will hear all kinds of price comparisons between organic and conventional food. It's said that you can pay anything from 10 to 50 percent more for organic food. It all depends how and where you buy—so let's look at some of the significant ways you can save money while buying decent and organic food.

1. COUPONS

Until recently, I confess, I always felt embarrassed using coupons at the store—I think its partly because of the impatient toe tapping that would go on in the line behind me as the often-confused cashier would unravel the tattered piece of paper that I had fished out from the bottom of my purse. I always seemed to get the confused cashier who would then make a huge drama of clipping out the relevant coupon while also having to check with the store manager—all that to save twenty-five cents off a four-dollar bottle of something. So for a long while, I just never bothered and watched in horror as my grocery bills got bigger. I could also rarely find coupons for things I wanted—especially Gorgeously Green items. I'm happy to report that things have changed and that you can start cutting and downloading coupons for all kinds of organic foods. Here are some good ones:

www.wildharvest.com
www.organicvalley.com
www.stonyfieldfarm.com
www.mambosprouts.com
www.littlecrowfoods.com
www.equalexchange.com
www.shopnatureoasis.com
www.scojuice.com

I think we'll keep seeing more and more organic companies offering coupons, so go to www.gorgeouslygreen.com/coupons to find the latest and greatest offers.

Also check in your newspaper supplements. They are beginning to do a few organic coupons, and especially check in the front of any health food store you go to. If they don't have them, you can ask the manager if and when they'll be coming in.

2. BUY LESS

I know this sounds incredibly obvious, but the statistics on waste in this country are astounding. Twelve percent of all food bought for home use is never used, and according to a survey reported by the Texas Cooperative Extension Agency, 25 percent of edible food (in households, restaurants, stores, production) in the United States goes to waste. Here are the main reasons that we typically waste foods:

- We bought something for a particular recipe and never got around to making it.
- We bought something on special offer that we didn't really want.
- We bought a bunch of stuff in bulk and found we didn't need it or it moved past its sell-by date before we got to it.
- We just bought too much!

I have a rotating cupboard that has recently been cleaned of odd and exotic Eastern ingredients that are way past their sell-by date. I have nasty plastic bottles rattling around in drawers full of ghastly looking sprinkles from Lola's birthday parties way back, and I keep staring at a red tube of marzipan that I bought for a holiday recipe four years ago.

I'm also guilty of buying way too much. I think this stems from a fear that we'll run out—"better to be safe than sorry" sort of thinking. I'm learning my lesson quickly because I can't afford to waste any more food. Here's what I try to do:

- If a recipe calls for an unusual ingredient, I buy it only if I absolutely *know* that I will be using it within the next week and/or multiple times.
- I try an ingredient that I've never tried before at someone else's house before buying it, hating it, and tossing it.
- I buy in bulk only if I know I will use up the ingredients within a month or if I'm splitting the shop with a friend.
- I buy smaller packages of dried and canned foods, because in surveys it was found that a huge percentage of food waste was in this and the bulk-buying categories. On my pantry purge, I have to admit that I found two large bags of whole-wheat flour that were past their sell-by date and a large bag of sugar that was so hard, I couldn't even hack a knife into it.

My dear father serves as a brilliant example of how *not* to shop! He's had many hobbies over the years and gets a little obsessive about the latest thing that's piqued his interest—they say the apple doesn't fall too far from the tree! One of these "interests" was Chinese cooking—so off he went to buy sauces, bottles, and jars of the most foul-looking ingredients from a very peculiar Chinese store that he'd found online. As if this wasn't enough, specialized woks began to appear in my mother's overcrowded kitchen, not to mention an entire new knife collection for cutting raw fish! We were subjected to one rather unpleasant meal, and that was that. The wok, bamboo steaming baskets, and tins of lotus root got put up in the attic along with the Italian pasta machine from a few months earlier.

My husband will tell you that he "knows where I got *it* from"—but I remind him that my Gorgeously Green-ness overrides my compulsion for novel and exciting. I just have to make sure that my passion for a newfangled experiment is tempered with sound eco-friendly judgment. A good case in point is my new bread maker, which makes delicious bread—I was encouraged to buy a mini version so we would avoid any waste, but I now have to make upward of three loaves a week for my dear husband and daughter, who can't get enough of the irritatingly tiny seven-grain loaves.

3. COMPARE PRICES

Again, this seems a bit obvious, but it's worth the effort. Keep a budget book (a small recycled notebook from Staples works) and write down the items that you always buy: milk, bread, eggs, potatoes, tofu, chicken, and so on, and then write the price down after each major shop—this way you can keep track of price changes. This is especially important at large grocery stores because they tend to lure you in with the promise of lower prices across the board, but if you really keep track of their prices on certain items, you will be shocked at how they fluctuate. These stores assume that you won't be keeping a budget book—most people don't. Also take your budget book to other grocery stores and compare the prices of their organic items. There are huge disparities.

4. LIVE ON THE EDGE

Grocery stores are set out so that all the perishable foods are on the perimeter. When you realize that the biggest price markups are always on convenience, packaged, and processed foods in the store's inner aisles, staying on the outer edges of the store will encourage you to stick with the more cost-effective and eco-friendly foods.

5. BRANDED

Try to stick with the store brands (generic) since they are always cheaper. Also let go of some of your brand loyalty: Many of us habitually reach for a certain brand because it's what we've been led by advertisers to trust. If you compare the ingredients, however, there is typically no difference at all. Be sure to check out the large grocery chain brands of organic food. Some of these stores are Whole Foods, Publix, Trader Joe's, Safeway, ShopRite, Vons, Wal-Mart, and Kroger.

6. BULK BINS

Buying cereals, grains, dried fruit, beans, nuts, and legumes from the bulk bins will always save you a great deal of money and has the added eco-bonus of saving on the packaging, too.

7. GOING SOLO

It helps to shop alone rather than with your partner and particularly with kids. Whenever I take Lola along, it's a disaster unless I pretend that I'm her rather fierce schoolteacher (notice I have to pretend to be someone other than the pushover mom that I am!). She wants this and that and leads me totally astray, as does my curious husband. I'm much better off on a solo mission.

8. STICK TO THE LIST

This is the toughest for me because I get very easily distracted by goodies and interesting-looking new things. The key for me is that I don't allow myself to pick up anything unless it's on my list. Sometimes, I think, "Ooh, what is that interesting-looking jar or packet?" and then ten minutes later, I'm all over it, checking out ingredients and deciding that we absolutely *need* it. So I have to stick to my list at all costs. Otherwise, I'll pay for it in more ways than one, not the least of which is getting home and my husband finding that we already have six of a similar product in the pantry.

9. BUY LESS MEAT

This is probably the most important one because organic meat and dairy are considerably more expensive than their conventional counterparts. I only buy grass-fed or organic meat, and so the price can be double that of the mass-produced variety. So that I can still afford it, I buy it just occasionally. I make it stretch further by buying cuts I can make into stews, or ground meat that I can use a little of in pasta sauces. I would rather eat humanely reared meat, with no antibiotics and hormones, once every two weeks than eat the other kind every day—better for my health and my pocketbook.

We also eat way too much meat as a nation. For our skinny jeans, our health, and our eco-impact, it makes sense to cut down considerably.

10. UNCUT VEGGIES

Instead of buying mini carrots, buy large uncut, un-peeled carrots, and you'll get more carrot for your buck! Never buy cut-up vegetables in a bag, because it's way more expensive and it's not much of a time saver anyway. The stalks of broccoli and cauliflower can be used in soups and pasta, and the rest can be converted into valuable fertilizer in your compost bin.

11. FRESH PRODUCE IN SEASON—OTHERWISE, ORGANIC FROZEN

Buying asparagus, green beans, and bell peppers in the winter will cost you a lot more, especially if they're organic. When they're not in season, instead buy spinach, green beans, corn, asparagus, peas, succotash, and berries frozen and organic.

CHEAPER CHICKEN

If you love organic chicken, here's how to keep the cost down:

- Buying a whole chicken is the most cost-effective way to go. If you don't know how to cut it up, you can ask your butcher at the meat counter to do it for you. If there is no one at the meat counter, go to www .gorgeously green.com and see my "how to cut up a chicken" video.
- Chicken thighs are delicious and are way less expensive than chicken breasts.
- Whole chicken legs are the third-best choice.

If you ever see jars of marinated bell peppers or sun-dried tomatoes on sale, grab a few for your pantry. They'll keep for a long time and are superhandy in the winter.

12. BUY CANNED FISH INSTEAD OF FRESH

Fresh fish tends to jack up the price of a weekly shopping trip. The healthy fish that are packed with omega-3s (wild salmon and sardines) are great to buy canned, especially if you are adding them to salads, pastas, and sandwiches.

13. LOOK FOR BARGAINS

I'm always on the lookout for a good bargain, and there are many to be had in grocery stores. When the store has overordered or just hasn't sold a particular item, it has to go on sale. If you go to a grocery store that doesn't have much organic food, you will see, ironically, many of their organic items (especially dairy) on sale. Start finding the stores that often have things on sale. You can also look for specials online. I regularly go to the Whole Foods site to see what they have on offer in my local store. Go to www.wholefoodsmarket.com/products/specials/index.html and type in your zip code—then pick your store and find out what's on sale. Some of the large grocery store chains have their own exclusive organic lines—items of which are often on sale.

14. STICK TO YOUR EATING PLAN

An eating plan always saves me money because it helps me make a comprehensive list that I have to stick to. If I know what the week's menus are, I can plan accordingly, making sure I've substituted seasonal recipes where I need to.

Also make a point of frequenting your produce or farmer's market toward the end of the summer season because they have a glut of fruit they need to get rid of—a golden opportunity for you to grab a few pounds of peaches, plums, or figs that you can make into preserves and jellies to last the entire year. A good time of day to go to the farmer's market is when they are about to pack up: Oftentimes the farmers don't want to haul back what they came to sell, and it will probably spoil in a few days anyway, so they will give it to you for next to nothing!

ORGANIC CUISINE FOR LESS THAN THE PRICE OF A BURGER KING MEAL

I used to think that it was okay for people who could afford to shop in health stores to eat organically, but what about the family of five who doesn't have the time or money to go anywhere other than a fast-food burger joint and get what's on offer? I decided to do a bit of research, convinced that I could cook a large, organic dinner for a family of five for *less* than a Burger King meal. I took myself off to the burger joint and did my calculations based on each member of the family having a large burger, large fries, and a drink.

I then went shopping for a good, healthy, delicious meal, and here's what I came up with: Tuscan Chicken Stew—serves five. It came in at six dollars under the fast-food bill.

I also can't accept the argument about not having time, because this meal takes ten minutes to prepare in a slow cooker, and if you can't afford a slow cooker, there are plenty to be found on the Web sites www.craigslist.org or www.freecycle.org or in thrift stores.

This stew is infinitely more nutritious, kinder on the planet, and less expensive than fast food—so if anyone gives you the "all right for those who can afford it" argument, give them the following recipe—and there's lots more where this one came from.

TUSCAN CHICKEN STEW

All of the following ingredients should be organic.

1 large yellow onion
2 leeks or 1 head of celery
4 carrots
1 vegetable bouillon cube
1 quart boiling water
1 large can whole tomatoes
8 chicken thighs (approx 2 lbs)
1 cup pearl barley
Pinch of mixed dry herbs
Sea salt and freshly ground pepper to taste

Chop the onion, leeks or celery, and carrots and place in a slow cooker. Dissolve the bouillon cube in the boiling water in a measuring cup and add to the slow cooker. Mix everything around, then add the remaining ingredients. Set the cooker on low heat and cook for 5 to 8 hours, then smell the gorgeous aroma filling your home when you return from work.

For other affordable recipes, check out the recipe section in this book. Most of them are designed to be in the same price range as the above recipe.

PRIORITES

Americans spend a smaller percentage of their income on food than Europeans do, and I would hasten to add that, on average, Europeans are healthier in the diet department. This may come as a shock to many of us, who think that food is horribly expensive and cannot fathom how on earth we're going to be able to afford *any* meat, much less grass-fed meat. It's all about prioritizing: The best-quality food I can find is essential for me because of health—I just don't want to be old, sickly, and hobbling around regretting that I didn't take care of myself better when I was able. I just think about all the useless things I can cut out so that I'll be able to afford meat that's reared without chemicals—just letting go of a few extra cable channels I never watch, a landline phone I never use, and three of the five coffee shop trips that I take weekly puts the extra cash in my account that's needed for good-quality food. Think about the little things that you can start cutting back on to make beautiful food affordable.

PULLING YOUR BELT IN

If you stop eating out and start cooking in, you will make the biggest money savings of all, plus you will undoubtedly lose weight.

If you think about how much a meal now costs at a restaurant, even a supposedly inexpensive one, it's pretty outrageous. It's hard to get a decent home delivery (and I'm not talking greasy pizza or MSG Chinese) for under the cost of a T-shirt—so, all in all, if you want to hang on to a wad of cash, get yourself and your partner into the kitchen and whip out your pots and pans.

Eating out a lot entails a lot of hidden calories, too—there's no telling how much cheap fat or oil was used, even if you go for clean and simple options like grilled chicken or fish.

The other thing that horrifies me about home deliveries, drive-throughs, and take-out food is the amount and kind of packaging involved. Most restaurants wouldn't dream of using sustainable or eco-friendly packaging because it's way too expensive—so polystyrene and plastic utensils still fly out the door and end up in a landfill, along with all the food that we didn't manage to force down from the over-size portions we were served. Let's get a grip and say no to costly, fat-laden food and waste—its just common sense.

CHAPTER TWELVE

From Scratch

Cooking from scratch is one of the biggest money-saving changes you can make. That extra bit of effort will pay off handsomely in a healthy body and wallet.

Nowadays, it's almost considered abnormal and terribly virtuous to cook things from scratch. What does "from scratch" actually mean? Instead of buying a premade soup, pasta, or meat dish (fresh or frozen), you buy all the individual ingredients as whole foods and prepare them from their raw beginnings. It's not rocket science or even hard to cook things from scratch. My husband and I do it almost every day and it's the most healthy and satisfying thing you can learn to do. I want to lure all you Gorgeously Green girls and your families back into the kitchen because the greenest (and I mean deep emerald greenest) thing you can do is to cook your own meals from real food.

Baking your own cookies, muffins, and even granola is very easy and is much cheaper than buying packets, boxes, or mixes. Homemade soups aren't even comparable to canned or pre-prepared soups in taste and quality, and take just minutes to prepare. Stews and casseroles can be made from scratch in a slow cooker, saving you time and money. The list goes on. Have a look at Chapter Fourteen, "Making Your Own."

The most important aspect of spending time in the kitchen cooking is that it brings family and friends together. Whenever I cook a meal, my daughter loves to be involved. We've had some of our most precious conversations over a mixing bowl or while topping and tailing green beans. What a gift for the people you love to have them come home to the aroma of a bubbling stew or freshly baked bread. When I'm panicked that I don't have time to cook, I remind myself that my grandmother raised four children and ran a pig farm, a chicken coop, and a huge garden while still finding time to cook three beautiful meals a day. I have a tendency to look back with rose-colored spectacles, and I'm sure my grandmother would have loved the convenience of packaged food occasionally, but still, there's something wrong if I can't carve out the odd twenty minutes here and there to prepare something that didn't come out of a box. The most important ingredient in all of these home-cooked dishes is love. There is nothing more satisfying than seeing friends and family greedily scraping a plate clean. I recently came home late from a particularly trying business trip that included sitting for hours in crowded airports. When I opened the front door, a delicious buttery aroma filled my nostrils and made my shoulders drop. My husband had spent hours preparing a vegetable pot pie (my favorite) from scratch. It was such a loving gesture, especially since it was his first ever attempt at making pastry!

Every culture has traditional foods that you can probably remember your grandmother making. Many of us have traveled far from our cultural roots and so have stopped eating those "real" foods that underpinned our existence. These were the recipes that were passed down from generation to generation—recipes that certainly weren't dreamed up by a man in a lab coat. If you examine the traditional foods of your culture, you'll find that they are healthy, whole foods that provided the perfect nutrients for where your people lived. I still hanker after some of the dishes that I remember both my English and my Scandanavian grandmothers cooked and then passed on to my parents. I hope that I can keep even a tiny part of these traditions alive for Lola. The only hope I have of doing that is by getting into the kitchen.

CHAPTER THIRTEEN

Your Eco-Kitchen

What is a Gorgeously Green Kitchen? It's a kitchen that is geared toward healthy living and leaving the lightest eco-impact possible. The two big issues here are making your kitchen more energy efficient and making it nontoxic. Let's deal with energy first.

ENERGY EFFICIENCY

The chances are that you use way more energy than you need to. Even if you don't believe that reducing your energy use will have any significant impact on global warming, you are probably a little miffed by your outrageously high energy bills. It makes sense to conserve whenever we can. I know that energy conservation is one of the most boring topics and, goodness knows, we've been blasted with energy-saving tips galore over the past couple of years—so let's just go over the essentials.

Your fridge-freezer is the SUV of your kitchen. It weighs in as the third-hugest energy guzzler of the home (furnace and AC rank higher), so it behooves you to make sure you're getting the best performance from the model you have.

We all know that Energy Star appliances are the way to go. Good for you if you've got one. But some of us are stuck with monsters from yesteryear and we have to make do. The best models, which mine isn't, are the ones that have the fridge on top of the freezer, so if you are in the market for a new one, make sure it has this setup. Side-by-side models use 20 percent more energy. Also, if you can, find one without the frost-free technology, because it uses 45 percent less energy. Follow these tips:

BEAUTIFUL COILS

Keep your coils shiny so your poor fridge doesn't have to work so hard and thus use more energy.

- Pull your fridge away from the wall and unplug it. If it's a built-in model, turn it off at the circuit breaker.
- Remove the coil cover panel (usually located at the bottom front of the fridge). It may just lift off or you might need to unscrew it. Older models have exposed coils on the back of the fridge.
- Use the long, narrow vacuum attachment and suck out all that nasty dust and debris.

- Make sure that it's not next to your oven. The heat from the oven will make the compressor work harder and use 25 percent more energy.
- Buy a fridge thermometer and make sure that it reads no higher than 38–40°F.
- Check the seal and get it replaced if it's looking like it's seen better days.
- Vacuum the coils every three months.
- Make sure you have only one fridge-freezer in operation. Many families keep a second one in the garage. Turn it off.
- Keep your fridge well stocked; it takes more energy to cool an empty fridge.
- Keep your freezer well stocked for the same reason, and if you don't have enough food to fill it, simply fill two liter bottles three-quarters full of water and stash them on one of the shelves.

What about saving energy in other areas of the kitchen?

- Gas is more efficient than electricity, so better to boil your tea kettle on the hob than to plug it in.
- If you've got the oven on, try to cook as many things as you can with that valuable heat (i.e., make a batch of granola while the chicken or tofu is baking).
- *Always* boil a pan of water with the lid on.
- Never stand chatting with the fridge door open while you decide what to pull out for dinner.

CONSERVATION

Water is becoming a very scarce commodity, so we need to conserve every drop we can. Here's how I save water in the kitchen:

- Boil and steam at the same time: potatoes and pasta below and green beans in the steamer above—it saves energy, too.
- Let the water from your boiled and steamed veggies cool and then use it to water houseplants or plants in your yard.
- Throw used food that cannot be composted into the trash rather than into the garbage disposal, which is very water and energy wasteful.
- Run the dishwasher only when full—energy saving, too.

WASTE AWAY!

I cannot talk about an eco-kitchen without mentioning composting. It is unequivocally the best way of getting rid of food waste. Having tried and tested virtually every composting model on the market, I highly recommend a compost bin called The Garden Gourmet (www.gardengourmet.com) if you have a yard. It's a monster black bin that will just swallow all of your fruit and veggie waste. All you need to do is to make sure you layer the waste with "brown matter," which can be dry leaves, dirt, wood chips, or sawdust. Also turn the compost with a garden fork or a long stick once a week, and if your climate is very dry, throw a gallon of water on it every once in a while to keep it moist. Every six months, you can lift up the hatch and take out bucketfuls of odorless, precious compost to put on your yard.

I also recommend getting a cute compost crock for your kitchen counter. You can add bits and pieces of waste as you go along and empty it every couple of days. I

ECO-IMPACT OF MY DISHWASHER

You'll be relieved to hear that for the most part, it's more eco-friendly to use your dishwasher (providing it's full) than to hand wash. A dishwasher will typically use half the energy, one-sixth the water, and a lot less soap than hand washing.

As the Gorgeously Green Diet involves a lot more cooking at home, there will also be a lot more washing up. Don't be afraid of loading your dishwasher up to the max with pots, pans, mixing bowls, wooden spoons, and the rest. If you run your dishwasher daily, pop your dishwashing brush and sponge onto the top rack (to sanitize) and add ½ cup of white vinegar to the rinse cup weekly. I also spray the Gorgeously Green All-Purpose Spray (page 166) all over the inside of the machine once a week.

have a white ceramic model from www.realgoods.com that has a carbon filter in the lid to keep out any odor.

If you live in an apartment or don't have a yard, I highly recommend The Bokashi Kitchen Compost Bin. You fill this kitchen-friendly bin with all your produce waste and add a scoop of the Bokashi powder, which speeds up the composting process so that you have odorless brown "gold" in half the time of a regular outside compost bin. You can purchase one at www.pottingbenches.com. You could also consider the Nature Mill automatic/indoor (www.naturemill.com) composting machine, which can live inside. It will speedily compost your waste as it heats and turns it every few hours—you'll hear some rather alarming grinding and chomping sounds coming from it! You need to add a lot of baking soda and sawdust pellets to prevent odor. The manufacturers say you can put in meat and fish, but I would tread carefully on that one because of the smell.

If you live in a duplex or apartment with a communal yard, ask your neighbors if they will share a compost bin with you. I cannot tell you how great it feels not to have to shovel all that waste into the trash. If you don't have a garden or any potted plants, find a nearby community garden by visiting www.pottingbenches.com or find out if any local schools have community gardens. Anyone with a yard or a garden will be really grateful for your compost.

GADGETS

I'm a total sucker for gadgets and have to be held back at every turn. Most of the ones that I rushed out and bought on a whim over the years ended up in thrift stores along with hundreds of others—cappuccino frothing devices, mini–food processors, and decorating kits, to name but a few. There are, however, a few gadgets that have remained firm favorites over the years and are, I am happy to report, also very eco-friendly, despite my husband's claim that "it would be a lot greener if we just made do with what we already have."

Bread Maker

I'm in love with my bread maker because:

- It uses very little energy.
- It bakes the most scrumptious bread.

- It saves me on all the packaging involved in regular bread.
- It saves me throwing bread away, since I only make a mini loaf when I need it.
- It enables me to make the exact kind that I want: organic, rye, millet, even spelt.
- It costs on average a dollar and a half for a beautiful, organic loaf, whereas in the store, it'll cost at least double that.
- The smell of freshly baked bread is one of life's great pleasures.

Yogurt Maker

I'm in love with my yogurt maker because:

- It uses very little energy.
- It allows me to make lactose-free yogurt.
- It makes the most scrumptious yogurt imaginable.
- It allows me to eat yogurt without any additives, including sugar.
- It avoids the numerous plastic pots that only sometimes get recycled.
- I get to feel like super-eco-mom every time I take the glass jar out.
- Is there anything better than a yogurt parfait made with organic berries and homemade granola?

Immersion Blender

I'm in love with my immersion blender because:

- It allows me to blend soups without having to transfer to a blender.
- It's superquick.
- It's really easy to clean.

I recommend the KitchenAid Immersion Blender at www.target.com.

Stainless Steel Kitchen Tongs

I'm in love with my tongs because:

- They can be used for literally everything.
- A day doesn't go by that I don't use them.

- Every decent chef uses them constantly.
- They're cheap—pick up a pair for less than ten bucks!

Mandoline Slicer (Kitchen Utensil for Cutting and Slicing)

I'm in love with this slicer because:

- I can slice all my fruits and veggies with ease.
- It makes a perfect chopped salad.
- It's fantastic for stir-frying.
- It requires only my own energy!

Bamboo Salad Spinner

I'm in love with this spinner because:

- It's made of bamboo, which is a renewable resource.
- It doubles as a salad bowl, which saves on washing up.
- It looks beautiful.

Toaster Oven

I'm in love with my toaster oven because:

- It uses only up to half the energy that a regular oven does.
- I can cook a whole meal in it.
- I can safely defrost food in it.

COOKING

PANS

So what is the most healthy and eco-friendly pan? There are two issues with pans. The first is the very controversial issue of Teflonlike nonstick pans that some say contain a chemical compound called polytetrafluoroethylene (PTFE) that, when heated at a high temperature, can kill a bird and affect a human's health. It should be noted that apparently Teflon will break down and release these chemicals only if it's heated beyond 300 degrees F. However, the last time I grilled chicken, my pan got up to 450 degrees F before the chicken even hit the pan.

The second is the issue of aluminum, which some feel is best to avoid because it can migrate into the food, leading to neurological changes in the brain and gradual deterioration, and could be part of the cause of Alzheimer's disease. You can switch to good old stainless steel or try out some of my favorite eco-friendly choices:

- COPPER FUSION—This is the crème de la crème of cookware. It is made primarily of copper, so the heat distribution is unprecedented. It's the favorite of many chefs and, because the line contains no aluminum whatsoever, you don't need to give leaching or flavor interruption a second thought. As if this wasn't enough, these pans are so sexy that you'll want them on display. They come in two or three different colors and are my firm favorite. See www.chantal.com.

- ANODIZED ALUMINUM COOKWARE—This is a great choice because the anodizing process locks in the cookware's base metal, aluminum, so that it can't get into your food. It is scratch-resistant and nonstick and heats evenly. See www.cuisinart.com.

- CAST-IRON COOKWARE—This is another great choice and can be good for you because a tiny amount of iron will migrate into your food—so great for women who are still having periods. Find bargain cast iron in flea markets and thrift shops; it keeps forever. You have to "season" it to avoid food sticking, but this is very easy to do.

- ENAMEL COOKWARE—If you like the heaviness of cast iron but can't be bothered with having to season it, you could go for enamel cookware, which is great for stews, sauces, soups, grains, etc. A Dutch oven is a large, cast-iron cooking pot with an enamel lining. They are great for making soups and stews. My favorite company for Dutch ovens is www .lodgemfg.com.

- CLAY COOKWARE—I love clay cookware because it is easy to use and great for a weight-loss diet since you really don't need to add any oil for cooking. You can also cook an entire meal in it and serve out of one of the decorative models. See www.romertopfonline.com.

If you are getting rid of Teflon pans, I suggest you call your local sanitation department to see if your curbside recycling program accepts old pots and pans. If your pans are in good condition, you may want to sell them on eBay or take them to your local thrift store.

UTENSILS

It would be a good idea to switch all your plastic utensils—spoons, spatulas, knives, and measuring spoons—for either stainless steel or bamboo. Plastic can leach bisphenol A (BPA, a hormone-disrupting chemical) into food, especially when it gets hot. I love the entire line of Chantal stainless steel utensils (www.chantal.com) and I like to use bamboo salad servers and mixing spoons (www.greenfeet.com).

COOKING TECHNIQUES

There may be healthier ways of cooking and preparing your food than you currently employ—let's look at the effects on our food of these different techniques:

Zero cooking/raw food: This has got to be the healthiest way to go because the digestive enzymes, vitamins, minerals, and antioxidants remain completely intact. I love raw food and eat a huge raw salad almost every day, though I enjoy cooked food too much to become a raw foodie.

Steaming: This is the next best thing to raw, provided you *lightly* steam your food. Make sure you take your veggies off the heat before they are ready, for they will continue to cook after you take them off the heat.

Steam-frying: This is healthy and great for a weight-loss diet because instead of using oil to fry, you simply substitute a little chicken or vegetable broth. Use the broth as you would the oil, by heating it in the pan and then adding the food. I recommend steam-frying meat, fish, and veggies whenever possible.

Frying: Frying with oils is not the healthiest way to go because a high heat not only destroys the nutrients in the oil but can also cause the formation of free radicals. Every oil has a "smoke point," which is the temperature it can be heated to without burning. See "Best Oil Choices" (page 41).

Barbecuing: You should use great caution when cooking out. Studies have shown that women eating a lot of char-grilled foods have a twofold greater breast-cancer risk than women who never ate these kinds of foods. Charred foods can create compounds (mutagens) that have been linked to cancer. Fatty drippings from meat and fish can splash onto the coals and create carcinogenic compounds, which are returned to the food via the smoke—a very nasty thought. Studies have shown that adding the herb rosemary can help because it's packed with free-radical-fighting compounds, which can aid in blocking the dangerous compounds from forming. A great way to use rosemary is to add it to marinades and also sprinkle a few leaves over whatever you cook. Rosemary is delicious with lamb, chicken, and fish. Also make sure you:

- Trim excess fat off red meats before grilling.
- Marinate the meat/fish away from the grill to avoid a sudden burst of flame.
- Never char your foods.
- Don't cook directly over the flames. Moving the food to the outside of the grill is safer.
- Grill your chicken with the skin, as it acts as a protective cover, and then remove the skin before eating.
- Never cook frozen meat on the grill as the outside will char and the inside will remain underdone.

CLEANING

The air quality in our homes can be seven to ten times worse than the air quality outside. This is due to a plethora of toxic chemicals that we unwittingly bring into our homes. One of the worst offenders is cleaning supplies. I highly recommend that you switch to eco-friendly alternatives. Make sure you have the following ingredients handy. They clean almost everything:

- Food-grade hydrogen peroxide—Best germ buster on the market. It's inexpensive and easily available from drugstores and grocery chains.

- White vinegar mixed with hot water is the perfect window cleaner and can be used for a variety of other cleaning chores, too.
- Baking soda is great for scrubbing tough stains or wooden cutting boards, tubs, and sinks.

GORGEOUSLY GREEN ALL-PURPOSE SPRAY

This is a great spray since the essential oils are antibacterial and leave a wonderful scent.

32-ounce sprayer bottle (opaque is best)
2 cups water
2 cups white vinegar
20 drops of tea-tree oil
1 drop of lavender essential oil

Simply pour all the ingredients into the sprayer and use for everything from kitchen counters to tables and fridges. I also recommend spraying down your counters once a week with food-grade hydrogen peroxide. It's the best ever germ buster. Put some in an opaque sprayer (as it's light sensitive), spray, and wipe with a clean, damp cloth.

What do you wipe down your sink sides with? My guess is paper towels. They are a convenience that is really hard to kick. I keep a roll handy for those nasty little jobs like scooping up tomato seeds from a cutting board, but for the most part I use old rags instead. I cut up old sheets, towels, and T-shirts and keep them in a hamper in my laundry room. I use one a day and toss it in a laundry pile with a bunch of other rags, which I clean once a week. I always buy recycled paper towels (www .marcal.com) since I can't bear the thought of more trees being cut down for the sole purpose of making my sink shiny.

I love the eco-friendly sponges made by Twist (www.twistclean.com), and all my dish towels are made from organic cotton.

STORAGE

I use glass or ceramic jars with airtight lids for storing cereals, grains, flours, and even cookies. It's a good idea to have a selection of different-size containers at the ready, since with your eating plan, you may be buying nuts, dried fruits, rice, and grains from bulk bins. You will find a great selection of storage jars and canisters at both www.bedbathandbeyond.com and www.crateandbarrel.com.

I always use glass to store food in my fridge. Warm food and plastic are not a good match because the chances of toxic chemicals leaching from the plastic are increased when it heats up. I have an excellent set of various-size glass containers with plastic lids from www.pyrex.com.

PACKAGING

It's really important to consider what your food is packaged in, not just because we want to avoid all the paper and plastic, but also because it's another way for toxins to seep into our food. Substances can actually migrate from aluminum foil, plastic wrap, aluminum cans, and takeout containers.

Even more scary is microwave and put-straight-in-the-oven packaging, which can transfer more of these toxins into your TV dinner. Polystyrene, still widely used in restaurant takeout food and cups, not only contributes to more than four billion pounds of trash a year but can also migrate styrene into your food or beverage. Styrene mimics estrogen in your body and can disrupt normal hormone function, contributing to thyroid problems and other hormone-related issues, including breast and prostate cancer. All this is another wonderful reason for staying away from prepackaged and processed food.

KNOW YOUR PLASTICS

PETE

THE NUMBER 1 WITH THREE ARROWS AROUND IT—PET OR PETE (POLYETHYLENE TEREPHTHALATE):
(a) Safe to drink out of ONCE, so do not reuse (b) Recyclable
Example: water bottles

HDPE

THE NUMBER 2 WITH THREE ARROWS AROUND IT—HDPE (HIGH-DENSITY POLYETHYLENE):

(a) Safe, but few are reusable, so best to avoid reusing altogether (b) Recyclable

Example: milk bottles

V

THE NUMBER 3 WITH THREE ARROWS AROUND IT—VINYL OR PVC (POLYVINYL CHLORIDE):

(a) AVOID—emits carcinogenic chemicals (b) Not recyclable

Examples: shampoo bottles, peanut butter jars

LDPE

THE NUMBER 4 WITH ARROWS AROUND IT—LDPE (LOW-DENSITY POLYETHYLENE):

(a) Safe (b) Recyclable BUT only at Whole Foods, Wal-Mart, and
plastic-bag recycling centers

Examples: bread and frozen food bags, most plastic wraps

PP

THE NUMBER 5 WITH THREE ARROWS AROUND IT—PP (POLYPROPYLENE):

(a) Safe (b) Recyclable BUT only with certain curbside recycling programs;
please check with your local sanitation department.

Examples: ketchup bottles, yogurt tubs

PS

THE NUMBER 6 WITH THREE ARROWS AROUND IT—PS (POLYSTYRENE):

(a) AVOID—can leach styrene, a possible human carcinogen (b) Recyclable BUT only
with certain curbside recycling programs; please check with your
local sanitation department

Examples: Styrofoam containers, take-out food containers, plastic cutlery

OTHER

THE NUMBER 7 WITH THREE ARROWS AROUND IT. INCLUDES VARIETIES:

1. PC (polycarbonate):

(a) QUESTIONABLE—composed of hormone-disrupting bisphenol A

(b) Not Recyclable

Examples: most plastic baby bottles, Nalgene brand and sports water bottles

2. PLA (polylactide):

(a) Safe (b) Not recyclable but can be composted

Examples: plastics made from renewable sources like sugarcane, corn, and potato starch

SHADES OF GREEN

LIGHT GREEN

Invest in one of the new eco-friendly pans (see page 163). Make sure that you have a
good set of sharp chopping knives and some reusable glass containers for storing your
chopped-up produce.

BRIGHT GREEN

Take a look at your entire pan collection and decide what has to go. Either invest in a
new set of pans (see page 163) or pick out one or two all-purpose pans to begin with.

Good choices are a large sauté pan and a stockpot. Consider buying a yogurt maker. I recommend the Yogourmet from www.lucyskitchenshop.com. The instructions on how to make the yogurt, and everything you need, including the starter cultures, will be shipped to you. It comes with one large plastic jar, so I suggest you order the large glass jar too and substitute. Alternatively, you can buy the Euro Cuisine Yogurt Maker from www.target.com. This comes with individual glass jars.

DEEP GREEN

Make sure you are cooking with *only* eco-friendly pots, pans, and utensils. Get rid of any plastic wrap or aluminum foil. Buy yourself a yogurt maker (www.lucyskitchen shop.com) and a sprout maker (www.wheatgrasskits.com).

I also suggest you get yourself a bread maker. If your budget is tight, check out your local thrift store or www.craigslist.org. They always have them!

I know this sounds insane, but if you have a yard, consider a chicken coop—you can buy adorable tiny ones from www.backyardfarms.com. The minute I have a decent-size yard (right now a pool takes up most of it), I'm going to keep three to four chickens. Just imagine going outside to get fresh eggs in the morning.

CHAPTER FOURTEEN

Making Your Own

"I can't cook!" is the war cry of thousands of women. But if you can read, you can cook. It's easy to follow a recipe. Even Lola, aged seven, is getting pretty good at it. Cooking is like riding a bicycle: You may topple over a couple of times, but once you've got the hang of it, your confidence will grow and, before you know it, you'll be doing wheelies—or soufflés!

The most important thing is to make sure you know the basics. Once you get the hang of the following recipes, you'll be in good shape because they form the base of so many dishes and/or are kitchen classics.

STEAM-FRYING ONIONS

Since many dinner recipes begin with frying onions and sometimes garlic, celery, and leeks, it's a good idea to learn to fry with broth instead of oil. This method is especially useful for soups and sauces. To get the full benefit of healthful oils that lend flavor to your dish (olive, walnut, and sesame), add 1 tsp of the oil after cooking.

- **2 tbsp chicken or vegetable broth**
- **1 onion, chopped**
- **2 garlic cloves, finely chopped**

Place the broth in a skillet on a high heat until it bubbles. Add the onion and stir. Cover the skillet. After 2 minutes, stir again. Steam for 1 more minute before stirring in the garlic. Steam-fry for 1 minute before you add the meat or fish or vegetable for the remaining recipe.

GHEE

Ghee is clarified butter and in Indian ayurvedic medicine (the oldest health care system in the world, which is now being used extensively in complementary medicine) it's considered to have great healing properties, including being good for your joints and your skin. It's delicious on toast, baked potatoes, eggs, or whatever you would normally put butter on. I love that it's always easy to spread because you can keep it at room temperature without its spoiling. It's easy to make. All you need is:

1 16-ounce box of organic butter

Place the butter in a heavy saucepan on the lowest heat possible. Let it bubble and simmer for about 30 minutes. Keep checking; you can tell it's ready when there are white curds floating on the top and brown granules on the bottom of the pan. Be really careful that it doesn't burn. As soon as you see the brown bits on the bottom of the pan, remove from the heat.

Allow it to cool for 5 minutes and then pour it through some unbleached cheese-cloth (available at Whole Foods) into a glass measuring cup. You can then pour it into an old jelly jar or glass container with a lid. It'll keep for up to a month at room temperature.

CREAMY MASH

I love mashed potatoes with almost everything—it's the ultimate comfort food. I have added some cauliflower so you will get the added nutrients from this wonder veggie, plus it makes it really tasty.

Serves 4
2 extra-large or 4 medium potatoes cut into ½-inch slices
1 small cauliflower head, cut up
1 tbsp butter
½ cup milk
Sea salt and freshly ground black pepper

Simply boil the potatoes and cauliflower in a large saucepan of salted water until tender. Be careful not to overcook or the potatoes will disintegrate!

Drain and mash well and stir in the butter and milk until creamy. Season and serve.

SUPER-SIMPLE STOCK

I cook with a lot of stock because it's tasty and it's a healthy substitute to use instead of oils and fats. It's so easy to make and freeze that I strongly suggest you give it a go. It also uses up leftovers.

4 cups filtered water
1 yellow onion, peeled and cut in half
1 carrot
1 stalk celery, coarsely chopped
1 bay leaf
3 sprigs fresh parsley (optional)
½ tsp mixed dried Italian herbs
Salt and freshly ground pepper

Simply put all the ingredients in a stainless steel saucepan and bring it to a boil. Turn down the heat and simmer for 30 minutes. Remove from the heat, cool, then pour into ice cube trays (for easy-to-use cubes) or a safe plastic container. When it has completely cooled, freeze. It will keep up to 3 months in the freezer.

CHICKEN STOCK

When I tell people I use homemade chicken stock in soups or risottos, they are so impressed. I don't let on how easy it is.

Make the supersimple stock as above, but add a chicken carcass. It's a great idea to make this after you've cooked and eaten a roast chicken. Keep the giblets in the fridge and add them to the pot, too. Turn the heat down low and gently simmer for two hours. Voilà!

WHITE (BÉCHAMEL) SAUCE

This is a must-know recipe for every Gorgeously Green Girl because it's so very easy and is used for a multitude of dishes,

STOCK-FREEZING TIP

I love to store my stock in ice cube trays because I can then take out one or two cubes for steam-frying or to add to a soup. Because I'm wary of leaching plastics, I have discovered the perfect solution, called Baby Cubes (www.babycubes.com). They are made of safe plastic, are an ideal size, and come with little lids.

If you've made a large quantity of stock, when it's cool, skim off the fat and then you can pour it into a gallon-size plastic freezer bag placed inside a medium-size bowl. Keep the bag of stock in the bowl until it has frozen and then remove the bowl. When you come to defrost it, it'll fit perfectly into the bowl.

from lasagna to vegetable gratins and chicken pot pies. I learned to make it when I was about ten and have already taught Lola how to do it.

1 tbsp butter
1 tbsp whole-wheat flour
2 cups milk
1 cup vegetable stock
1 tsp Dijon mustard
Sea salt and freshly cracked pepper

Melt the butter over a low heat in a medium saucepan. Add the flour and mix it with the butter until it forms a little ball. Add ½ cup of the milk and stir—the key is to *keep stirring* the whole time. If you get any lumps, take it off the heat and beat with a whisk or wooden spoon until lumps disappear. As the sauce quickly thickens, add some more milk and keep stirring. Keep adding the milk until it's all used, and then add the vegetable stock. Bring to a boil, then reduce the heat and simmer for 5 minutes. Stir in the mustard and salt and pepper to taste.

You can turn the béchamel into a cheesy sauce by adding 1 cup grated sharp cheddar or Parmesan cheese at the end.

EASY ALL-PURPOSE TOMATO SAUCE

So, so easy and mega-useful, add it to pasta, pizza, meat, egg, or fish recipes. In summer, use fresh tomatoes; in winter, use canned organic tomatoes. Better still, in the summer, when there is a glut of tomatoes, make two enormous stockpots of this sauce and freeze it in individual glass containers or freezer bags (plastic, I know—but we can't be perfect all the time)—that way you'll be set for the winter months.

6 to 8 large tomatoes or a 22-ounce can organic whole tomatoes
2 tbsp olive oil
3 large cloves garlic, chopped
2 tbsp tomato purée
1 tsp sugar
Small handful chopped fresh basil or 2 tsp dried basil
Salt and freshly ground black pepper to taste

To skin fresh tomatoes, make a few slits in the skin and place them in a deep bowl. Cover them with boiling water for 1 minute, then remove from the water. Hold them with a towel to prevent burning your fingers and slide off their skins. Chop the tomatoes.

Heat the olive oil in a large skillet over medium heat. Add the garlic and cook for 2 minutes or so without coloring (or steam-fry—see page 164). Add everything else and mash with a wooden spoon. Simmer for 15 minutes, and that's it!

OLD-FASHIONED MAYO

The risk of salmonella poisoning from raw egg is virtually nil if you are using organic eggs—so worry not!

- **1 large egg yolk**
- **1 teaspoon Dijon mustard**
- **Juice of 1/2 lemon**
- **3 cups olive oil**
- **Sea salt and freshly ground black pepper**

You can use either an electric whisk or a food processor (the food processor works only if you are making a large batch, with at least 4 eggs—unless you have a mini–food processor). Take the eggs out of the fridge a couple of hours before you need them. All the ingredients work better at room temperature.

Start by whisking the egg, mustard, and 1 tsp lemon juice. While you're whisking, *very slowly* add 2 tablespoons of the olive oil a tiny bit at a time. If all is well and the mixture hasn't separated, begin to add the rest of the oil in a very thin, continuous stream. The key with mayo is that you don't want it to "separate." If it does (you can tell because it'll look lumpy and weird instead of creamy), you can try adding 1 tbsp boiling water. If that doesn't do the trick, you'll have to start again and add the separated batch to the good batch.

Once all the oil is blended, add the rest of the lemon juice and then store in the fridge until you're ready to use it.

EASY BREAD

You can bake a loaf of bread as follows in a few easy steps. Alternatively, you can sling all the ingredients into a bread maker and go watch TV or meditate. The process of hand making the bread is very therapeutic for me, so on a bad day, I whip out my loaf pan and indulge in this soothing activity.

> ¾ cup warm water
> 1 package active dry yeast
> 1 tsp salt
> 1½ tsp sugar
> 1 tbsp butter, softened
> ½ cup whole milk
> 3 cups all-purpose or bread flour

Pour the warm water into a large bowl. Slowly stir in the yeast until it's dissolved. Stir in the salt, sugar, butter, and milk. Mix in 2 cups of the flour. Add a little more flour, 1 tablespoon at a time, until the dough forms a ball.

Turn the dough onto a floured board and knead (dig your fists in and twist them around repeatedly for 2 minutes). Add more flour as needed to prevent the dough from becoming sticky. Place the dough in a greased bowl. Cover the bowl with a kitchen towel and leave it in a warm spot for 45 minutes.

Preheat the oven to 375°F.

Form the dough into a loaf shape and place it into a greased loaf pan. Let it sit for 30 minutes.

Place in the center of the oven and bake for 45 minutes, or until you see a light brown crust.

CRISPY COCONUT AND FLAX PROTEIN BARS

These are my favorite bars/snack because they contain every nutrient I need for optimal health and they are simply delicious. It's a good idea to spend some time gathering the ingredients that I recommend, because once you have them, you'll be able to make quite a few batches. The brown puffed rice is sold by www.naturespath.com in bulk, so it's very budget friendly. You will also find this brand at most health food stores.

> Yields 10–12 bars
> 4 tbsp virgin coconut oil★ (www.spectrumorganics.com or www
> .tropicaltraditions.com)
> 4 tbsp brown rice barley syrup (www.lundberg.com)
> 1 tbsp agave syrup

1 tsp vanilla essence
2 cups puffed brown rice
2 tbsp ground flaxseed
1 tbsp shredded coconut
2 scoops whey or hemp protein powder
2 tsp cinnamon

Preheat oven to 325°F.

Melt the coconut oil, brown rice syrup, agave syrup, and vanilla in a small saucepan over a low heat until liquefied. Mix all the other ingredients together in a large bowl. Add the syrup mixture and combine really well, making sure that each puff of rice is coated. Press into a nine-inch-by-nine-inch baking pan and place in the center of the oven for 10 to 12 minutes until it is bubbling. Remove and cut into bars before it cools.

*NOTE: It is a huge misconception that this oil will raise your cholesterol or make you fat. It's actually one of the healthiest oils that you can eat because it's full of a fatty acid called lauric acid, which is an antimicrobial agent. Therefore, it can protect you from pathogens, bacteria, and viruses. It also contains caprylic acid, which is very effective in treating *Candida* and other yeast/fungal problems.

MIRACULOUS CHOCOLATE MACAROONS

This is the ultimate sweet treat that is actually good for you. These are ridiculously easy to bake, so enjoy!

6 egg whites
¼ tsp sea salt
½ cup agave nectar
1 tbsp vanilla extract
3 cups shredded coconut
1 tbsp unsweetened cocoa powder

Preheat oven to 325°F.

In a mixing bowl, whisk egg whites and salt until stiff. Fold in agave, vanilla, coconut, and cocoa powder. Drop the mixture onto a parchment-lined baking sheet, one rounded tablespoonful at a time. Pinch each macaroon at the top.

Bake for 10–15 minutes, until lightly browned.

SECTION FOUR
Growing Your Own

CHAPTER FIFTEEN

Creating a Garden

A great way to reconnect with our food source is to grow it. If you try to grow any kind of vegetable, you will gain a wonderful understanding of just what it takes to sustain our food system. I invite you to pull on a pair of gardening gloves and start right away. Whether you live in a tiny city apartment or a mansion in the middle of nowhere, you are going to love growing your own. The most positive thing about growing your own food is that is guarantees your food security. It's heartening for me to realize that even in the case of severe food shortages, I would be able to put a decent amount of food on the table from my garden. As food prices continue to rise, there is going to be a resurgence of urban gardening.

During wartime, both here in the United States and in the United Kingdom, citizens across the nation rolled up their sleeves and planted "Victory" gardens. They used any spare space they could get their hands on: vacant lots, scrubby backyards, and even apartment-building rooftops. It's amazing to realize that in the United States they produced 40 percent of all the vegetable produce consumed in the country. Victory gardening was considered a morale booster that made citizens feel empowered by contributing their labor, and they felt rewarded by the produce grown. With oil prices unstable and our food security increasingly uncertain, I think it's equally critical that we come together as a nation now and do what we can to grow our own. In the summer, you can save up to 40 percent on your weekly produce bill by growing the vegetables you eat the most of. In the winter, you can save up to 20 percent.

What exactly you can grow each month will depend very much on your local climate. However, if you're crafty, you'll always be able to grow *something* year-round. Use row covers, cold frames, and greenhouses—where there's a will there's a way! Here's a very general idea of what you may, depending on your climate, be able to eat from your garden seasonally:

Spring: artichokes, asparagus, broccoli, green beans, spinach, strawberries, sweet corn, chard, and watercress

Summer: beets, bell peppers, blueberries, cantaloupe, cherries, cucumbers, figs, grapes, green beans, lima beans, pole or bush beans, okra, peaches, plums, radishes, strawberries, corn, summer squash, tomatoes, watermelon, zucchini, basil, rosemary, oregano, and sage

Winter: apples, Brussels sprouts, kale, pears, persimmons, and sweet potatoes

Year-round: cabbage, carrots, celery, cauliflower, lettuce, onions, potatoes, and turnips

CONTAINER GROWING

It's amazing what you can do in a very small space. I have two small raised beds in my backyard and an enormous variety of containers. I use hanging baskets, terra-cotta planters in every size, old coffee cans, wooden barrels, even a hollowed-out stump of a wind-felled trunk I found on a beach. I grow enough produce to keep us going in the summer and enough to supplement our diet in the winter. I always grow as many herbs as I can, since they are very expensive to buy from the store, and this way I can just pick what we need.

Second to cooking, gardening is my most therapeutic activity. I can stomp into my yard in a foul temper, and after only ten minutes of weeding, pruning, and watering, I'm a different person. If you would love to learn to meditate but find it hard to sit on a cushion staring at a wall, just try a bit of gardening—just by virtue of tending a plant, you'll swiftly move into the present—your thoughts centering on the tiny job at hand. Meditating is simply the process of slowing down your thoughts.

If you are unused to gardening, take tiny steps to begin with so you don't get overwhelmed and then discouraged. Your plants are like small children—they need a lot of care and attention, especially when they are starting out. Because, as an organic gardener, you are not going to be adding any "inputs" in the form of chemical herbicides and pesticides into your garden, it requires a little more effort and ingenuity to keep the pests at bay—however, once you've got the hang of it, you'll be thrilled.

I suggest that beginners start with a small planter or tub and plant an easy salad seed. A great choice would be either a mesclun mix (also called gourmet salad mix or baby spring mix) or arugula (roquette). Both of these organic seed mixes can be ordered from www.seedsofchange.com. Since baby salad leaves are delicate, they don't like extreme cold or heat, so early spring is the ideal time for sowing, depending on where you live. If your climate is relatively temperate most of the time, you may be able to grow them year-round. You will be lessening your eco-impact considerably by growing your own salad greens because you'll be cutting back on packaging and food miles.

Here are a few easy steps to growing your own gourmet salad:

1. Pick out a planter or a tub. It should be at least a foot high.
2. Place your container in a spot that gets at least four hours of sun a day.
3. Fill the container with organic potting soil.
4. Sprinkle the seeds thinly and evenly across the soil and then cover with a thin (one-eighth inch) layer of soil. Water with a gentle sprinkler nozzle on your watering can.
5. Make sure you water regularly, and remember that shallow window boxes dry out really quickly, especially when it's hot. You may have to water them twice a day.
6. Harvest the leaves when they are about three to four inches tall. You can cut them with a pair of scissors, leaving a one-inch stub.
7. Water the stubs with a solution of diluted fish emulsion. I like Lilly Miller Alaska Fish Emulsion, which you can find at Ace Hardware (www.acehardwaresuperstore.com) and many good nurseries. It'll encourage new growth and you should be able to get two or three harvests out of the original seeds.

During the winter months, you may want to consider growing your herbs and salad leaves in an indoor kitchen garden called an AeroGrow (www.aerogrow.com). This is a small countertop growing machine that uses a highly oxygenated growing chamber, water, and artificial light to grow your plants. I love mine because I am addicted to fresh basil and love that I can make fresh pesto all winter long. You can grow herbs, salad leaves, tomatoes, and even flowers in your AeroGrow. Although I prefer my plants to be grown in good, real soil because they will draw up all the nutrients they need out of the soil, it's a great compromise for the winter.

RAISED BEDS

If you have a patio or yard, you may want to consider building some raised beds. They can be any size you choose and are typically rectangular. You build them with just four planks of wood from your local hardware store. In my experience, raised beds produce the best vegetables that I've ever managed to grow. Regardless of the quality of the soil in your backyard, with a raised bed you can begin from scratch, making sure your plants will have the best possible start. I highly recommend getting the book *The Vegetable Gardener's Bible* by Edward C. Smith (Storey Books). Mr. Smith shows you, by the use of easy-to-follow color photographs, exactly how to construct a raised bed. I could never be described as a DIY diva, and yet Mr. Smith had me shooting off to the hardware store, measurements in hand, and schlepping home with my planks. In just one hour, I managed to assemble and hammer the whole thing together. Another couple of hours and I had been to and returned from the local nursery with eight heavy bags of potting soil, and by lunch the whole thing was completed. As I hungrily sank my teeth into a grilled veggie sandwich, I realized that a morning of hard physical labor had been just the thing to lift me out of the rather bleak mood I'd woken up in. As I chomped away, I gazed at my masterpiece and imaged the baskets of fresh, colorful produce that I'd be harvesting in just a few months.

THE SOIL

Successful gardening is all about the soil. Soil is one of the planet's most valuable resources—without it, we wouldn't be able to eat. Conventional farming has devastated topsoil all over the world, so as powerful consumers who vote for organic farming with our dollars, we are helping to protect the very thing that we depend on for life. Soil is the earth's skin. However, the topsoil, which is only about a foot deep, is what gardeners and farmers are most concerned with because it is the nutrient-rich layer of soil that can be easily damaged by environmental pollutants. Healthy soil is like a healthy body—it will protect the plant against disease. This is why good soil needs to be your first priority. Even if you are caring for a simple houseplant, it's worth repotting it with nutrient-packed organic potting soil so that your plant will thrive for years. If you don't, after a few months, a rather sad-looking plant may be heading to the compost pile.

Food plants need a lot of nutrients, and so when they've finished growing, your soil will need replenishing before the next plants go in. The best way of doing this, rather than buying expensive bags of organic fertilizer, is to compost. This is why I'm obsessed with putting all my old food scraps to good use. I adore that I can just chuck them into the big monster bin and six months later I have an abundance of one of the most precious fertilizers on earth. If we could all compost—individually, in our neighborhoods, communities, businesses, and schools, we could and would make a huge difference. If you have even a small yard or live in an apartment, you can get started right away.

If you don't compost, you'll need to make sure that you use a good, organic fertilizer every month. Visit your local hardware store or nursery and you should be able to find an organic fertilizer specifically for fruits and vegetables. These fertilizers are in powder or liquid form and have to be diluted with water. Read the package directions carefully because the amount to use can widely vary.

CHAPTER SIXTEEN

Composting

$\mathscr{I}$ have tried every conceivable composting device on the market and my all-time favorites are:

THE GARDEN GOURMET

This is a large black bin—not the most attractive thing in the world, but well worth it—and you can probably hide it behind a fence or some bushes. You'll also need an occasional box of composting enzymes (speeds up the process) and an old rake or pitchfork to turn over the compost once every two weeks.

All you have to do is layer your waste (old fruits, veggies, breads, pasta, even paper) with brown matter (yard clippings, old leaves, dirt, etc.). Think: garbage lasagna! The layers help the whole pile stay oxygenated and you need the oxygen to break down the matter. Finally, make sure the whole pile stays reasonably moist—if you live in a really dry area as I do, throw on a bucket of water weekly and that should do it.

See www.gardengourmet.com.

WORM COMPOSTING

I do adore my worm bin. For those of you who didn't see it, the worm bin was set up incorrectly when I was demonstrating it to Oprah on her show, and all the worms crawled out all over the set! She was pretty freaked out—not a big worm fan. But these little pink critters make the best compost imaginable. The Can-O-Worms is a worm composting bin, which is brilliant because it's a stacking system. That is, once the worms are done eating all the waste on one level, they crawl up to the next level, leaving you free to whisk the old level away and use all the wonderfully nitrogen-rich compost on your plants. Worm bins are great if you have limited space, and they are perfect for any of you who don't have a yard. The bin doesn't smell at all, so if you can get over having worms in your kitchen and have someone to donate the compost to, an apartment dweller can get rid of all their veggie scraps in this delight-ful way!

See www.unclejim.com.

CHAPTER SEVENTEEN

Plan of Action

THE FOUNDATION

Whether you have chosen to create raised beds or use your own existing garden beds, how can you make sure that your plants will have the best possible start? If you have new raised beds, filled with organic potting soil, you may want to add some compost or a bag of worm castings. You can buy worm castings from a nursery. This is soil that has been aerated by the worms and is nitrogen-rich, which is an important nutrient for your plants.

If you are starting off with existing soil in your yard, I highly recommend testing your soil with a little testing kit. I remember visiting the "Eco-Home" in Los Angeles—an old craftsman home in Los Angeles owned by a visionary lady with a wise and gorgeously green twinkle in her eye. I was bowled over by her garden. Right in the middle of the city, in a relatively small backyard, she had everything edible growing that you could imagine. On closer inspection, these plants were thriving. On a hot fall day, when my tomato harvest had come to an end and I had virtually nothing else growing, this garden was a cornucopia of delicious produce. The secret was her soil, and she explained to me how you can't expect a healthy, happy plant without healthy, happy soil. Just as I can't thrive on a diet of junk food, a plant can't thrive in barren soil. She was all for the soil test kit, primarily to test the pH of the soil. I recommend one called the Rapitest Soil pH Test Kit from www.heirloomseeds.com, which will tell you if your soil is too acidic or too alkaline. Most garden soils have a pH of between 4.0 and 8.0, and vegetables that you want to grow will do best with a soil pH of between 6.0 and 7.0.

FIXING IT

If your soil isn't the perfect pH, you can easily fix the situation by adding either limestone for too-acidic soils or organic matter (pine needles, brown leaves, or sawdust) for soils that are too alkaline. Fall is the best time of year to add these amendments. You should be able to buy limestone from your local nursery, and you can also take the results of your soil test there and see if they recommend any other amendments.

PLANTING

Deciding what to grow and what plants to put next to each other is really important in an organic garden, as many "companion" plants and herbs act as insect repellents.

Companion plants are plants that work well together to repel specific pests. For example, garlic and onions repel many pests because they are stinky, and marigolds planted around tomatoes help repel the destructive nematode. Check out the companion chart on http://gardenersnet.com/atoz/compan.htm.

Also, think about what you and your family really love to eat. In the summer, we can't get enough tomatoes, so I plant loads of them; we like a bit of zucchini—not too much, so I put in only two plants. Consult with your family and ask them what they would like to grow. It's a great gift to involve smaller members of the family. Although weeding wasn't my favorite chore as a child, the reward came with the picking. I learned so much from just hanging around watching my mom in the garden, and I hope to pass some of this on to Lola.

MULCHING

The final important step for your organic garden is to add a layer of mulch, which will help protect the soil, conserve water, and stop too many weeds from growing. You can use old grass clippings, pine straw, hay, or wood chips as mulch. Pack it all around your plants and they'll be good to go.

IRRIGATION

Since water is now such a scarce resource, I advise spending time to find out the most efficient ways to water your plants. If you can have someone help you before you prepare your soil, you could save a lot of money. There are some fantastic devices available at your hardware store—the best is probably a drip irrigation system, which is like a hose with tiny holes in it that is set underground near the roots of your plants. This will eliminate water waste from evaporation.

HARVESTING

It's so thrilling to peek under the leaves and see your first cucumber or zucchini of the season. I was almost delirious when I sent Lola down to the garden to pick a handful of strawberries to put on her yogurt. It had been quite a feat to protect the succulent little berries from greedy birds, but we'd managed! One summer, I harvested so many tomatoes that I gave bags away to everyone I knew. I also made gallons of tomato sauce that I stashed in the freezer. They kept us going in pasta sauces for the whole winter. You'll learn by trial and error, and the big lesson comes at harvesttime. What thrived? What languished, and what did you get too much of? It's a great idea to keep a little gardening journal. You can dig it out in the spring and remind yourself what to plant this year.

YOUR PLAN OF ACTION

LIGHT GREEN GIRL'S PLAN

If you are a complete novice, I suggest you start with a planter or a window box. You can either order one from www.plantcontainers.com or you can pick one up from your local nursery. I prefer a planter because it's deeper and so won't need to be watered so much. You could also try a hanging basket, particularly if you have very little outside space.

Your task is to plant an herb garden in your planter or window box. Pick out the herbs that you will use the most. My suggestions for what will work well with the eating plan are:

Summer: parsley, oregano, thyme, sage, basil, cilantro, and rosemary
Winter: chives, parsley, and dill

These can all go in one planter. In another planter (and you can use any large old container; yard sales are great places to find old planters), plant some mint, for it needs to be by itself. If you plant mint in a planter or garden, it will spread and strangle the roots of your other plants and herbs.

If you already have an herb garden, start out with sowing some salad leaves. A mesclun mix or arugula are my favorites. You can plant them in a large planter, window box, or raised bed. Make sure the seeds and potting soil are organic.

You can mail-order your seeds from www.organicaseeds.com.

BRIGHT GREEN GIRL'S PLAN

You are going to attempt to grow something that you love to eat. If you are relatively new to gardening, stick with the plants you are familiar with and don't get too ambitious. I got ahead of myself last year and tried all kinds of exotic veggies, and it was a disaster. I've learned that it's better to perfect what I know and not to introduce anything new unless I'm really prepared. Here are some suggestions that will work in beds, raised beds, or planters:

Summer: cherry tomatoes, zucchini, cucumbers, eggplants, bell peppers, chili peppers, and strawberries
Winter: chard, watercress, and kale

So choose two or three items to cultivate and put all your time and effort into raising them with as much care as you can. It's also worth having a planter of herbs near your kitchen (or on your kitchen windowsill) since organic herbs are expensive to buy and they totally transform your dishes into something wild and wonderful (see the eating plans).

DEEP GREEN GIRL'S PLAN

If you consider yourself the darker shade of green, it's time to pull those gloves on and discover how much food you can grow.

If you don't have the yard space, get online and find out if there is a community garden or small farm near you, where you can rent a plot on which to grow your garden. I highly recommend you buy yourself a copy of *How to Grow More Vegetables (than you ever thought possible on less land than you can imagine)* by John Jeavons. It will teach you everything you need to know about organic gardening.

I also recommend visiting www.communitygarden .org to find out if there are any existing community gardens in your neighborhood, or how you can start one.

If you have a decent-size yard—no excuse, girl. Get out there and start digging. Your garden can be your own personal gym/sanctuary, so you get three for the price of one: fitness, food, and peace.

Make sure you are growing as many herbs as you can. As a Deep Green Girl, you want to avoid any unnecessary trips to the store to buy plastic packets of herbs. Find a sunny windowsill and use a window box or even an old coffee can.

HERB TIPS

- If you have a lot of herbs that you can't use up, lay them on a baking sheet on the lowest possible heat in your oven. Leave them for half an hour or until dry and crispy. Remove the stalks and store in old herb/spice jars or resealable plastic bags.
- The best way to cut up parsley, cilantro, mint, and basil is to snip them with a pair of kitchen scissors into a glass.

SECTION FIVE

Fitness

CHAPTER EIGHTEEN

Get a Move On

SMART MOVES

The smartest, most feel-good thing you can do is to fire up a fitness routine to end all fitness routines. You've got to get moving if you want to live a longer, happier life, so you may as well jump in now and figure out a way to take your fitness to the next level. If going green means taking actions that have a positive impact on the environment—that must include your body, too. Numerous scientific studies have determined that regular exercise is a large part of preventive health care. According to a massive U.S. study of postmenopausal women, vigorous exercise can reduce the risk of breast cancer by 30 percent.

If you are a computer or couch diva and do the bare minimum in the exercise department, it's time to whip on some tennis shoes and get your limbs moving. If you want to shed even a *pound* of weight, you will not do it by diet or miracle pills alone. Sure you could stop eating altogether and become a limp and lifeless version of yourself, but the Gorgeously Green Diet is about nourishing and nurturing yourself. Life is way too short to be kidding yourself that you look fabulous with three percent body fat. Women with curves are sexy.

I feel fantastic when I exercise, and by "exercise" I mean breaking out into a sweat with my heart pounding. It staves off hunger and can turn a gray, depressing day into a jump-for-joy kind of day. I *never* initially feel like doing it—ever! I'll have my yoga mat out, weights at the ready, and I'll procrastinate like crazy, suddenly finding awful jobs like cleaning out the hamster's poop-filled bed, *anything* rather than picking up those weights. I've learned, however, if I simply make the first move onto the yoga mat, bicycle, treadmill, or even out the door for my walk, the mind will follow. I've learned over the years to get on with it, as avoidance is infinitely more painful.

Your fitness plan is as important as your eating plan, so it's time to start figuring out what you want to do. Some of you may be appalled at the thought of walking for even twenty minutes a day, and others of you may already be pounding the treadmill. The key is for every one of you to jack up your current fitness level. Training is called "training" because you are teaching your body to cope with a new challenge. If you found lifting ten-pound weights impossible a year ago but can now easily manage, it's time to increase the weight. If you can pound the elliptical on a ridiculously high level for more than an hour, without passing out, then your body has gotten used to that particular challenge and it's saying, "Huh, I'll just mellow out here 'cause I know this one backward." You've got to trick your body—keep it on its toes, give it something it's not used to. This may be why my stubborn friend Melinda keeps moaning about the fact that she cannot lose weight, even though she runs five miles a day on her treadmill. I keep telling her she should switch to cycling or intensive weight training, but she won't move out of her comfort zone. I invite you to move out of yours.

Another reason exercise is even more important than cutting down on calories is because, when you starve yourself, your metabolism slows right down. Your body is very smart and knows that it needs to conserve as much energy as it can. This is why breakfast is so important: It gives your body the message that it's going to be well taken care of in the food department—then it won't grab on to every calorie for dear life, storing it as fat. Remember that your entire system is geared toward getting and storing energy. Exercise boosts your metabolism and will help you gain a few pounds of gorgeous lean tissue as you lose the fat, which is why you should never weigh yourself, because muscle weighs more than fat. This precious lean tissue also helps metabolize the fat. Exercise also stops you from eating out of boredom.

REALITY CHECK

Look at the box below and write out exactly what exercise you do on each day of the week. Even if you do just a ten-minute dog walk daily, write it down so you can see where to go from here.

Monday	Morning	
	Afternoon	
Tuesday	Morning	
	Afternoon	
Wednesday	Morning	
	Afternoon	
Thursday	Morning	
	Afternoon	
Friday	Morning	
	Afternoon	
Saturday	Morning	
	Afternoon	
Sunday	Morning	
	Afternoon	

HOW MUCH?

Everyone is different, so it would be crazy to say that every man, woman, and child needs *X* amount of exercise weekly. What is obvious, however, is that we all need some kind of exercise *every day* unless we want to grow fat, infirm, or old before our time. This exercise doesn't have to be a leaping-up-and-down-and-running-five-miles affair either—it purely depends on your daily circumstances and fitness level. I think the most effective and fun way is to mix things up: I do something different almost every day of the week so I don't get bored. Here's an example of what I did last week:

Monday	Cycled to the grocery store and back (3 miles) and did 10 minutes of abs in front of the TV
Tuesday	1 hour of washing windows/scrubbing floors in the morning 1 hour of vigorous yard work in the afternoon
Wednesday	20 minutes on my rebounder and 10 minutes stretching afterward

Thursday	Practiced yoga for 30 minutes in the morning Took a 30-minute brisk walk to the store in the afternoon
Friday	Did a 40-minute aerobic/dance DVD at home with a friend
Saturday	Took a 45-minute hard hike with my husband
Sunday	Cycled to the farmer's market (2 miles total) and did a fun dance DVD with my daughter in the afternoon

So you can see that I break it up and often incorporate exercise into my daily activities. I don't think you should have to go to the gym to keep fit, so I'm going to show you how to do all the essentials at home. The most important thing is that your exercise is vigorous. Vigorous exercise could include demanding yardwork or housework, digging, chopping wood, running, fast jogging, fast walking (preferably on hills), tennis, and aerobics.

GOAL

My goal is to maintain my current weight and to build a bit more muscle and strength. What's yours? Think about it for a moment—do you want to lose a bunch of weight, do you want to lose a little weight, or are you happy with the way things are but concerned about your health and bone density?

In the box on the next page, write your goal and remember to write it in the present tense—as odd as that seems, it will become a reality if you do!

MY GOAL

I feel full of energy and superstrong. My abs are tight and my arms are defined, my seat is toned—dare I say "sculpted"—and I don't even know how much I weigh. It doesn't matter because I look and feel great. Oh, and my lower back isn't hurting anymore.

YOUR GOAL

THREE GORGEOUSLY GREEN FITNESS RULES

1. Do at least *one* vigorous exercise every single day.
2. Find something you love. Dance, tennis, trampoline—if you love it, you'll do it.
3. Find an exercise buddy—someone to hike or jog with, play tennis with, or meet up with to do DVDs a few times a week. If you work in an office, you could even organize a group to go power walking after lunch. The only thing required is a pair of decent sneakers, speaking of which, check out a fantastic fitness shoe called the "anti-shoe" (www.swiss masaius.com). They are made by a company called MBT and are designed to not only work your leg and bottom muscles 40 percent more than you would normally do while walking, but also completely correct your posture while standing. They are the perfect shoe for the office girl who is committed to pounding the sidewalks on a daily basis, as they

also considerably reduce your impact, thus taking care of your joints—important if you're walking on a hard surface.

GETTING THERE

How are you going to get superfit? If you are horribly inflexible—can't get anywhere near touching your toes sort of thing—flexibility will be a priority. If you get out of breath going up stairs, then cardio should be first on your list. If you see nothing but dangly bits when you look in the mirror, some weight training may be in order. Ideally, you want to balance all three aspects of your routine:

1. Flexibility
2. Strength
3. Aerobic

Just know that you don't have to do it all at once. The key is to carve out short amounts of time. A vigorous ten-minute hike or jog twice a day will do the trick if you're time challenged. Anyone can find ten minutes to do a bunch of squats and lunges—even if you have to do them in the bathroom at work! So let go of the notion that you have to schlep over to a sporting goods store and get kitted out in spandex for a routine that you'll never stick to. This is going to be an activity that you will work piecemeal into your everyday routine.

CHAPTER NINETEEN

The Exercises

EXERCISES FOR A SIMPLY GORGEOUS BODY

These are the exercises that will take care of every major muscle group in your body. They will help you to gain lean muscle tissue and melt away any unwelcome fat. They are really easy—they should only take you a couple of days to master—and you can pick and choose, depending on which area you want to work on.

STRENGTH

Here's where you build the strength you need for your everyday life: powerful abs to protect your back, strong arms for lifting all those boxes of designer shoes, killer thighs for—hmmm, you choose! And most important, strength training and all the exercises here will help to increase your bone density, which will help you to avoid the crippling effects of osteoporosis. So here we go.

UPPER-BODY ROUTINE

You can do this short routine at home. All you need is a pair of 2–5-pound weights (depending on your fitness level), an inexpensive set of bands,* and a chair.

---

*You can buy the bands at any sporting goods store, and Target has a great selection. You can buy them with or without handles, and different colors denote varying levels of difficulty. I recommend buying a pack of different colors. The handles are entirely up to you and make little difference to the exercises that follow.

1. Triceps Dips on a Chair *(for sexy and sculpted upper arms)*

You can do this exercise in your kitchen, living room, or office. It will strengthen and define your triceps.

Sit on a chair, placing your hands on the edge of the seat (as shown). Move your feet about 2½ feet away from the chair, with your knees bent at right angles. Keeping your bottom and your back as close to the seat as possible, dip your bottom as low as you can, and then raise it up to the level of the seat.

Repeat 10 times.

Pause.

Repeat 10 more times.

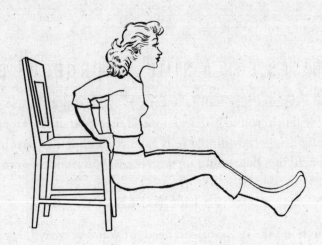

2. Push-Ups *(for a beautiful chest)*

You should practice these press-ups on a soft floor (carpet, rug, or yoga mat).

Get good at Version 1 before attempting Version 2.

VERSION 1:

Come down onto your hands and knees. Move your knees about 1 foot back from under your hips and cross your shins. Place your hands a little more than shoulder-width apart, turned slightly in toward each other with your fingers spread.

As you exhale, slowly lower your chest to the floor, and as you inhale, press yourself back up. Make sure you draw your stomach muscles in, keeping your core really firm as you perform your push-ups.

Repeat 10 times.

Pause.

Repeat 10 more times.

VERSION 2:

Come down to your hands and knees. Place your hands as in Version 1. Stretch your legs straight out behind you. Keeping your legs very straight, perform the push-up as you did in Version 1.

Repeat 10 times.

Pause.

Repeat 10 more times.

3. The Locust Pose (for strong back muscles and to open the chest)

This is a yoga pose, which is a safe and gentle way to strengthen the muscles alongside your spine.

Lie on your belly on a soft surface, with your feet together and your arms and toes stretching back. Your chin stays on the ground to begin with.

Turn your palms up and raise your arms parallel to the floor and stretch them back.

As you inhale, raise your chest, legs, and head as high as they can go without straining. Look forward and breathe evenly. Stay in the pose for 30 seconds, then release back to the floor, turning your head to one side.

Repeat 3 times.

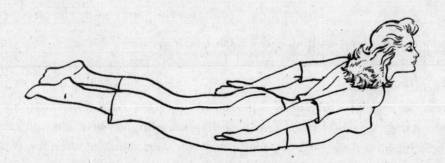

4. Biceps Curl *(for gorgeous, shapely biceps)*

Get out your bands. Bands come in varying tensions. You can decide which one to use, but the tension should be challenging. If you want to increase the tension to make this exercise more difficult, set your feet farther apart.

With your feet together, place the bands underneath your feet. Grip the ends of the bands and, keeping your elbows digging into your sides, draw your fists slowly up to your shoulders and then release down until your arms are straight.

Repeat 15 times.

Pause for 40 seconds.

Repeat more 15 times.

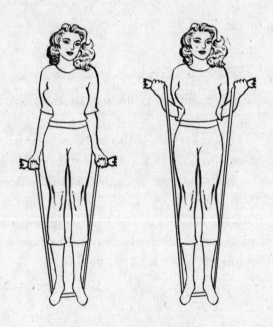

5. Shoulders *(for maintaining strong, shapely shoulders)*

OVERHEAD PRESSES:

This exercise makes for beautifully shaped shoulders. Try to do it at least twice a week.

Sit on the edge of a chair or stand with your knees slightly bent. Engage your abs and hold medium weights (2–5 pounds) just over your shoulders, keeping your elbows bent at right angles as if you were a goal post. Press your weights overhead.

Make sure you don't arch your back. Lower the weights back down until they are at ear level again.

   Repeat 12 times.

   Pause.

   Repeat 12 more times.

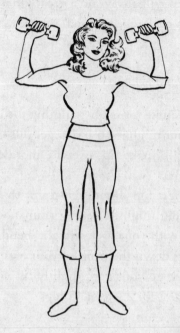

LATERAL RAISES FOR SHOULDERS:

This exercise targets a different part of the shoulder and is excellent if performed in conjunction with overhead presses.

   Hold light-to-medium weights (2–5 pounds) and, making sure your elbows are slightly bent, lift your arms out to the sides to shoulder level. Lower your arms back down until the weight brushes your thigh, then repeat. Try to perform 2 sets of 15 reps.

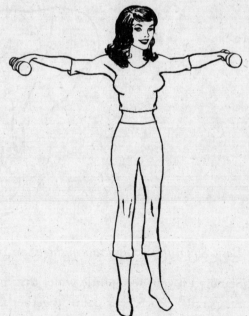

LOWER-BODY ROUTINE

Basic squats and lunges will always do a great job if you want to sculpt your bottom and thighs. Prepare to challenge yourself, for it's a small price to pay for those skinny jeans.

Dead Lifts (for a beautiful behind)

There isn't a better exercise for really sculpting the lower part of your bottom. It also targets the back of your thighs—so try to get this one down! It's worth investing in some heavier weights to make this exercise more effective. Ideally, work your way up to 10-pound weights.

Stand with your feet hip-distance apart, with medium-to-heavy weights (5–10 pounds) in front of your thighs. Keeping your shoulders back and your chest open, pull your abs in and, with your back straight, bend and fold forward from your hips and lower the weights down the front of your legs toward your lower shins. As you draw the weights back up your legs, slightly tilt your pelvis and squeeze the lower part of your seat. Repeat for 2 sets of 15 reps.

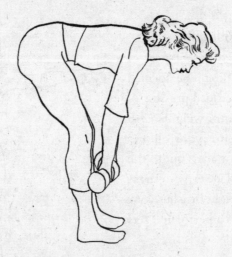

Basic Squat (for sexily sculpted thighs and behind)

Stand with your feet a little wider than hip-width apart, making sure that your feet are parallel. Place your palms together in a prayer position at your chest. Keeping your chest lifted, lower your sit bones all the way down until they are level with your knees. As you come back up, tense your bottom muscles.

Repeat 10 times.

Rest for 30 seconds.

Repeat 10 more times.

You can challenge yourself by performing a couple of sets while holding your weights on top of your shoulders.

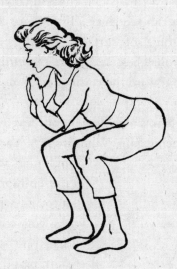

Basic Lunge (for firm and fabulous hips and thighs)

You can do your lunges anywhere and anytime. Plug into your iPod and imagine your tiny, sculpted tush in a bikini this summer.

Step your right foot out in front of you, making sure your shin and thigh are at a right angle. Lower your left knee down toward the floor.

Repeat 10 times.

Change legs and perform 10 reps.

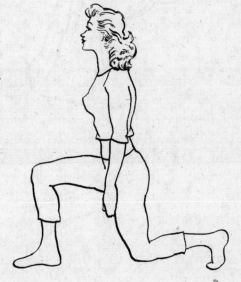

ABDOMINALS

There are an infinite number of really effective abdominal exercises you can do without any machines or gadgets. I highly recommend the three below.

Passing the Cushion or the Ball (for a lean and green tummy)

This exercise works very well with a couch cushion (any size will do) or an exercise ball. The exercise ball makes this sequence a little more challenging.

Lie down on your back on a soft surface, with the cushion or ball at your side. Draw your knees up into your chest and place the cushion or ball between your feet. Straighten your legs up toward the ceiling, gripping the cushion between your feet.

With straight arms and legs, slowly lower your feet and hands down toward the floor. As you inhale, raise them again. When your feet are directly above your hips, reach up with straight arms to grab the cushion and again lower straight legs and arms down toward the floor. As you come up again, when your arms are straight above your shoulders, pass the cushion to your feet, and then repeat the whole thing 10 more times.

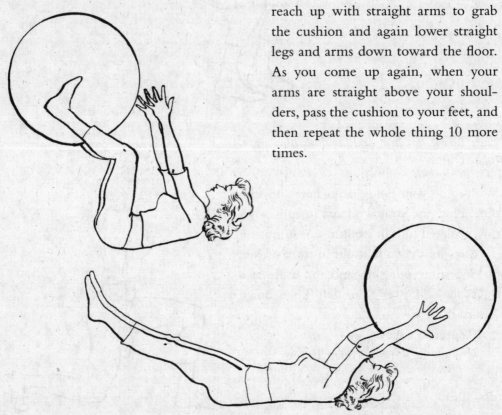

Chair or Ball Crunch 1 (for a rock-hard core)

Place a chair on a soft surface and lie down on the floor with your calves up on the seat of the chair or on your ball. Interlace your fingers behind your neck, taking your elbows out to the sides. As you exhale, raise your chest as high as you can toward your knees.

Repeat 15 times.

Rest for 30 seconds.

Repeat 15 more times.

Chair or Ball Crunch 2

You can vary Crunch 1 by taking one elbow to the opposite knee and then switching. You should repeat 10 times (a twist to either side qualifies as 1 time).

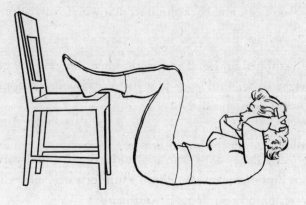

CARDIO

If you hate cardio, you can easily find a way of making it fun. I like to fit some heart-racing exercise into my busy day. Going to the gym isn't time effective for many of us, and remember that gyms tend not to be the most eco-friendly places on earth. A typical treadmill uses 1,500 watts of energy per hour, the equivalent of running your energy-guzzling fridge for three hours. You'll be burning fossil fuel rather than calories to get there, unless you walk, cycle, or run. Most gyms don't limit the use of towels, don't provide eco-friendly soaps and shampoos, and don't use chlorine filters or low-flow showerheads. There are a few green entrepreneurs who are attempting to create greener gyms. Some of these initiatives include passive solar designs, low VOC (volatile organic compound) paint, and energy-saving heating and cooling systems. Plans are also under way in different cities to create treadmills and bicycles that harness pedal/human power to create energy.

Combo

I love to do a combo workout of jogging/walking/lunges and squats. I jog for one or two blocks or until my heart rate gets high, and then I slow down to a fast-paced walk for another two blocks. I stop periodically and do a couple of sets of lunges and squats. It's really fun and less embarrassing (you can laugh at each other) if you do it with a friend.

If you are in a park, you might want to time your stretches of jogging/walking. You could start off with 3 minutes of jogging followed by 4 minutes of fast walking and then gradually increase. The lunges and squats will keep your heart rate up. Remember to do a good front and back thigh stretch when you're done.

FRONT THIGHS:

Stand with your feet together. Bend your right knee and grab the back of your right foot with your right hand. Pull your foot in toward your sit bone while drawing your tailbone forward. Switch sides.

BACK THIGHS:

Stand with your feet a little more than hip-width apart. Bend your knees and fold forward from your hips until you come into a full forward bend. Clasp your elbows. Gradually try to straighten your legs. If your hamstrings are tight, keep your knees bent. If you can straighten your legs, lift your kneecaps, firm the front of your thighs, and make sure your weight is evenly distributed between the balls of your feet and your heels.

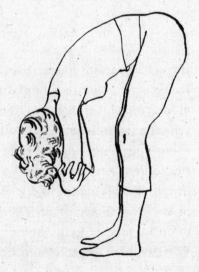

Rebounder

I love this mini-trampoline. A NASA study found it to be 68 percent more effective than jogging. You can buy fold-up models that come with a canvas carrier for you to take on the plane! I love that I can get up from my desk and do a quick ten-minute burst of aerobic exercise without having to even think about going outside. It is a zero-impact exercise, so is great for just about everyone, despite your age or ailments. I think it's one of the most effective and safest aerobic exercises around. Don't go for a cheap model, and be sure to invest in one that's really safe. The gold standard is Needak. It'll cost the same as a nice outfit, but it's a wonderful investment that will last you a lifetime.

Skipping Rope

I know this isn't going to be everyone's cup of tea, but it's an extremely good way of raising your heart rate quickly. Skipping is really *hard*! My daughter insisted that I try to beat her in jump rope the other day and I thought I was going to have a heart attack! No wonder boxers skip to keep in fighting form. If you have any injuries or a dodgy back, neck, or knees, I wouldn't recommend it. However, for the more sprightly among you, skipping is a supereffective aerobic exercise. And a basic skipping rope will cost you the price of a latte. You can get more fancy and expensive, but if you're just starting out, I recommend going with an inexpensive one.

Bicycle

Every Gorgeously Green Girl should own a bicycle. You can save up for a fancy one (www.electrabike.com—my personal favorite) or you can pick one up off eBay or Craigslist. The best thing is that it does double duty: exercise and errand transportation. I love grocery shopping on my bike. I have a large basket clipped on to the front and take a backpack, too. The ride back uphill is fantastic exercise!

Yard Work/Housework

When I get my teeth into my housework, I can easily break a sweat if I decide to do it at breakneck speed—which I do because I don't love it. Cleaning all my floors is a fitness workout level 12 if I want to make them shine. First the sweeping, then vacuuming, and then mopping/polishing, and by the time I've vacuumed the rest of the house, taken the trash out, emptied the compost bin, and hung out the laundry, I've definitely met my cardio criteria for the morning. Yard work can boost your fitness level considerably—so if you ever get the opportunity to dig and weed, grab it! My mother has never seen the inside of a gym or touched a piece of exercise equipment in her life, yet at the age of seventy, she puts most of us to shame with her physical stamina and energy, and it's all from yard work. She's out there every other day, pulling, digging, and hauling, and she says it doubles as meditation practice as well.

Walking

I love walking and wish I did it more, but living in urban Los Angeles doesn't inspire me the same way the countryside does. We can, however, walk anywhere. If you are stuck in an office all day, why not put on your tennis shoes and take ten to twenty minutes out to go for a really brisk walk. Do that twice a day and you'll have met your minimum exercise requirement. If I'm ever somewhere pretty or visiting a city, I just love walking—sometimes for hours, because it gives me a chance to air out my thoughts and to center myself. If I feel down, sluggish, or frustrated, a brisk—and I mean fast-paced walking with long strides for a good twenty minutes—usually does the trick. If you are lucky enough to live near steep hills, you've got it made, because you can move into a "training" zone for your heart. Same with hiking up hills or trails.

Swimming

I have to admit, I don't like swimming for exercise at all. It gets my heart rate going through the roof, but the very thought of having to get wet doesn't appeal. Frolicking around in the aqua water of the Caribbean is a different matter, but a chlorinated swimming pool—nah! That said, if you have access to a pool and don't mind getting wet, it's great aerobic exercise.

Exercise DVDs

I don't know why, but I always used to make fun of people who did home exercise DVDs, that is, until I met my friend Debbie, who has a killer body. When I asked her (as everyone does) how she got that shape—she told me she does a Jane Fonda DVD every single day and has done since it first came out as a video! I wasn't sure about the whole sweat-band-leg-warmer-high-impact thing, so I looked around and have found some incredibly effective exercise DVDs. My all-time favorite is *The Bar Method* (www.barmethod.com). This workout was designed by a ballet dancer and has you practicing tiny, isolated muscle contractions. It's very challenging, but you really do see very quick results. I also love Zumba (www.zumbafitness.com). This Latin American dance workout is a total blast as well as being supereffective.

FLEXIBILITY

I've been doing yoga for twenty years, so this is my sweet spot. However, if I don't practice regularly, flexibility can go as quickly as strength and cardio fitness.

It matters little whether you are a beginner or a full-on yogi; you still need to roll out a mat and do a few poses every week (or for some, every day). The joy of yoga for me is that, because it incorporates deep breathing, I find it incredibly relaxing and balancing. I'm sure my breathing is shallow, stressed-out breathing for most of the day, along with my shoulders being hunched up to my ears, so it only makes sense to take the time out to reverse some of the damage and to find a little patch of peace and calm in my chaotic day.

Here are the Gorgeously Green Essential Yoga poses that I strongly recommend you practice every week if possible—try five a day (hold each one for a minute only). You can easily practice them at the end of a walk or aerobic session. Always practice them when your muscles are warm.

1. Mountain Pose
2. Standing Forward Bend
3. Cobra
4. Down Dog
5. Triangle Pose
6. Warrior 2 Pose
7. Child's Pose
8. Bridge
9. Simple Twist
10. Thread Needle
11. Cobbler Pose
12. Legs Up the Wall Relaxation
13. Savasana (Deep Relaxation)

MOUNTAIN POSE

This is the blueprint for every other yoga pose and is an excellent opportunity to check your posture.

Stand with your feel together, arms down by your sides.

- Stretch and elongate your toes.
- Hug your leg muscles onto your leg bones, feeling the muscular energy.
- Point your tailbone down toward your heels.
- Lift your heart toward the sky and gently draw your shoulders back.
- Close your eyes and take 2 or 3 slow, deep breaths.

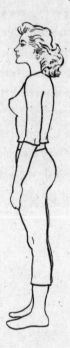

STANDING FORWARD BEND

To transition from the Mountain Pose, take your arms out to your sides and fold forward from your hips. Once in the pose:

- Bend your knees if you need to.
- If your legs are straight, lift your kneecaps.

COBRA

Slide forward from the Standing Forward Bend "butt in the air" pose into cobra.

- Slide your shoulder blades down and back, away from your ears.
- Press your tailbone down into the floor.

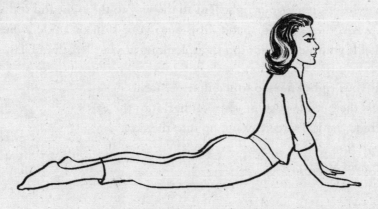

DOWN DOG

Use the muscles in your belly (yeah, right!) to haul yourself back into this pose.

- Spread your fingers.
- Draw your sit bones up and back.
- Draw your heels down toward the earth.

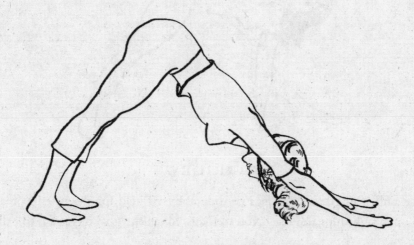

TRIANGLE POSE

This is a delicious pose that will strengthen your legs, open your hips, and lengthen your spine. It is a favorite of almost everyone I teach.

Stand with your feet 3½ feet apart and raise your arms out to the sides. Turn your right foot out 90 degrees and your left foot in 45 degrees.

As you exhale, stretch your right arm all the way to the right and really lengthen your right waist, then let your hand drop onto your shin or ankle (wherever feels comfortable). If your neck is not too tight, look up at your left thumbnail.

- Lift your right kneecap to stabilize the joint.
- Press the outside edge of your left heel into the earth.
- Extend the left fingertips up, up into the sky.

Switch sides and repeat.

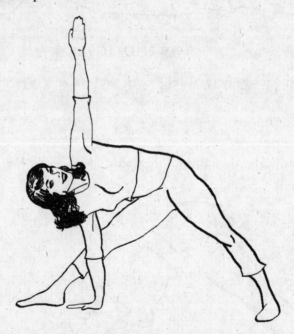

WARRIOR 2

This pose will strengthen your legs considerably—if held for the full 10 breaths, it will also open tight hips and teach you to focus. Since the goal of yoga is to calm and still the mind, this is a good pose to practice through simply observing the breath. Notice that when you get tired or fed up with holding the pose, your breathing will become more shallow and quicker. Train yourself to slow it down in the face of a challenge—it's a great lesson for everyday life.

Stand with your feet 3½ feet apart. Turn your right foot out 90 degrees and your left foot in 45 degrees. As you exhale, bend your right knee to a right angle, making sure the knee lines up with your middle toes. Extend your arms out to the sides, stretching through your fingertips.

- Push your right heel into the earth.
- Make sure that your right knee is directly above your right ankle.
- Gaze over your right fingertips.

Switch sides and repeat.

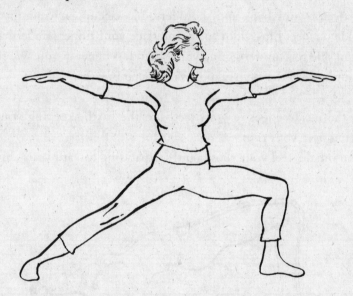

CHILD'S POSE

This is the most relaxing pose; it will open your hips and stretch out your lower back. If you've been sitting all day at the computer, it's a great pose to practice. Come onto your hands and knees, and take your knees a little farther than hip-width apart. Bring your big toes together and sink your sit bones down toward your heels. You can either have your arms outstretched in front of you or draw them down by your sides.

- Take deep elongated breaths to calm your mind.
- Draw your inner groin down toward the floor.
- Relax your jaw and your facial muscles.

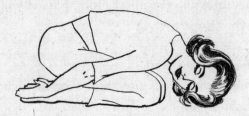

BRIDGE

This is fantastic for your back and shoulders. Lie faceup on your mat with your knees bent and your feet hip-width apart. Interlace your fingers underneath you and roll gently from side to side, wriggling your shoulders beneath you. While exhaling, lift your hips up toward the sky. Take 10 slow, deep breaths.

- Press the inside edges of your feet into the earth, keeping your knees pointing over your toes.
- As you inhale, feel your chest gently expanding toward your chin.

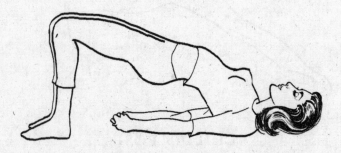

SIMPLE TWIST

This is a personal favorite that I practice whenever I am irritated, tense, or tired. Lie faceup on your mat with your knees drawn into your chest. Roll gently from side to side to massage your lower back. Let your knees drop toward your right elbow and spread your arms out in a T shape.

- Try to ease both shoulders into the earth.
- If your left shoulder is way off the floor, take your knees down lower.

Switch sides and repeat.

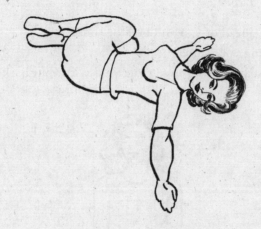

THREAD NEEDLE

If you suffer from tight shoulders and upper back, this is the pose for you. Start on your hands and knees. Thread your right arm under your left arm and slide your right arm across the floor all the way to the left until your right shoulder blade is resting on the floor. Take 5 slow breaths and then switch sides.

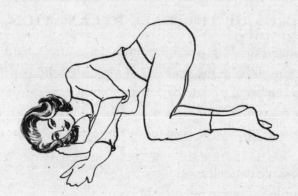

COBBLER POSE

This opens your inner groin muscles and is wonderfully relaxing to practice. Sit on your mat with your legs stretched out in front of you. Bend your knees out to the sides, bringing your heels in toward your pubic bone. Join the soles of your feet together. With your fingers, open the soles of your feet (as though you are opening a book). Now place your fingertips behind you on the floor and raise your hips, stretching your chest up toward the ceiling. Finally, clasp your fingers around your toes and straighten your back.

- Look straight ahead of you and breathe softly.
- Keep extending your spine.
- If you are unstable in this pose, practice it with your back against a wall.

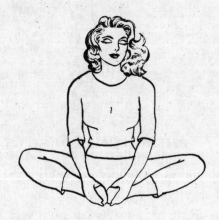

LEGS UP THE WALL RELAXATION

This is the best pose for tired legs and overall relaxation after a hard day. Sit sideways near a wall. Take your legs up the wall one at a time. At the same time, lever your body around so you are lying straight back with your sit bones against the wall. Draw your shoulders down, stretch your arms out to the sides with your palms up. Relax your feet and your face. Stay in the pose for 3–5 minutes with your eyes closed.

- Relax your facial muscles.
- Allow your breathing to be soft and even.

- When you are ready to come out of the pose, bend your knees and turn to one side before slowly coming up to a sitting position.

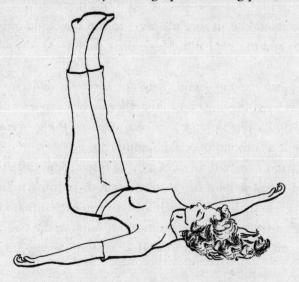

SAVASANA (DEEP RELAXATION)

If you can practice this pose just once every day, it will be a great gift. This is a powerful yet simple pose. Lie on your back on the floor with your arms and legs outstretched, your palms up. Your feet should be about hip-width apart and your arms a few inches from your sides. If your lower back is very tight, place a cushion or a rolled-up towel underneath your knees. Close your eyes.

- Release all your facial muscles.
- Breathe smoothly and evenly.
- Feel the energy pulsating through every cell of your body.
- Be still.

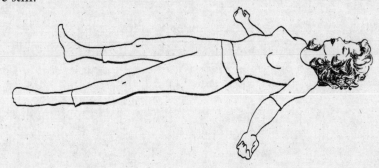

INSPIRE

Exercise, like eating, should be an absolute joy—to feel the blood pulsating through your body, to stretch and use your muscles to their fullest—this is what your body needs and wants.

If you are already an exercise fiend, why not inspire a reluctant friend to join you? Perhaps you can learn the yoga poses together or you can encourage your sedentary girlfriend to find a bicycle and join you to go to the grocery store. It sure takes the drudgery out of a monotonous shopping trip.

If, on the other hand, you're in need of a bit of inspiration, call up someone you know who practices yoga, or who has a good strength-training regime, and ask if you can join her for a few sessions—women love to help each other, so you won't be bothering anyone. Visit www.gorgeouslygreen.com and join the Green Fitness message board, where you can find support and chat with other Gorgeously Green Girls.

As you finish reading this chapter, get up right now and do one physical exercise to make you feel better. It starts with the first action—go take a walk, ride a bike, or try out one of the delicious yoga poses shown above. Just five or ten minutes could immeasurably change your day.

SECTION SIX

Beauty from the Inside Out

CHAPTER TWENTY

Healthy—Gorgeously Green

Gorgeous women are healthy from the inside out. It doesn't matter what age you are; if your entire system is in good working order and is being nourished by all the requisite vitamins and minerals, your skin, hair, and eyes will shine. As I grow older, I want to be healthier, stronger, and more vibrant. Gorgeousness is a quality of energy, and I've noticed that women who walk around with that glow are always the most gorgeous, regardless of their age or body shape.

The Gorgeously Green Diet is all about eating the healthiest foods on this planet—foods that are designed to nourish every system in your body. Foods in their natural state provide a veritable cornucopia of nutrients—everything we need to be in optimum health. I'm going to show you how to discover these beautifying foods, for there is clearly no point in slathering on expensive face creams if you're not taking care of the inside first.

ABSOLUTE ESSENTIALS

So what do we need to eat every day to be gorgeous? Do we need nutritional supplements? I think most of us need some kind of supplementation because even if we buy organic food, topsoil depletion and storage time greatly diminish the vital nutrients, and also the pollutants in our environment undoubtedly lead to a build-up of toxicity in our body. There are certain nutrients needed to support the functions of the organs that are directly involved in detoxification: the liver, the intestinal tract, and the kidneys—so let's take a brief look at the supplements that we should be taking on a daily basis. Keep in mind that this is a generic guide, and we all have different needs and challenges. Check with your doctor if you have specific problems. Nutritional supplementation should be customized to suit your specific needs. A thirty-year-old woman will need a set of supplements different from those of a fifty-year-old woman. Unless you are in tip-top health, I highly recommend going to see a nutritionist or naturopathic doctor, who can address your individual concerns about your age, hormonal balance, energy levels, sleep patterns, and overall health.

There are no supplements that can do a better job than eating fresh, organic food, but many of us just don't get the nutrients we need. The reasons for this include being a vegetarian or a vegan, not having access to fresh foods every day, and being overstressed physically and emotionally, which can impair digestion and absorption of vital nutrients.

RECOMMENDED DAILY PLAN

I am in pretty good health and eat a very healthy diet. However, I am always rushing and can easily stress myself out, which apparently affects my entire system.

Dr. Julia Tatum-Hunter, an internationally recognized dermatologist and the founder of Skin Fitness Plus in Beverly Hills, California, has shown that without inner health, everything you do on the outside works at only 50 percent, at best.

Dr. Hunter follows the recommendations of physicians and research from around the world, which has proved repeatedly that it's vital for women over the age of thirty-five to begin addressing their hormones, starting with the thyroid. Without replenishing the *essential* bio-identical hormones that our hectic lives deplete, it's very hard to preserve health, never mind beauty. A balanced endocrine system is of utmost importance to having health and beautiful, glowing skin. A balanced endocrine system also slows down the ticking of the clock.

Dr. Hunter has prescribed the following nutritional supplements for me. This is a generic plan that she prescribes to most of her patients, so it should work for you, too.

She constantly reminds me that stress increases production of the hormone cortisol, which is made in the adrenal glands, which sit on top of your kidneys. This makes you gain weight, particularly on your stomach and hips. So learning to manage and banish stress is a *very* useful skill! Nothing and no one is worth getting fat and sick for.

1. **Vitamins and minerals:** Everyone should get these in the form of green superfoods, and the more varied the ingredients the better—the more preferably organic, darker green, and sea vegetables you include, the better. The best thing you can do is to eat dark-colored antioxidant-rich fruits, healthy oils, and raw cacao. These foods are packed with *full* dosages of vitamins, minerals, and antioxidants from whole-food sources that preserve the ratio of one chemical to another, as they exist in the body. You can also take a vitamin and mineral supplement if you don't feel you are getting enough fresh produce. You get what you pay for, so make sure that you go for the best quality you can find. Dr. Hunter recommends Pure Synergy by the Synergy Company (www.thesynergy co.com) and Balance by CosMedix (www.cosmedix.com). I also like Realfood Organics Her Daily Nutrition by Country Life (www.coun tryLife.com).

2. **Super-antioxidants**—melatonin, CoQ10, and alpha-lipoic acid: Dr. Hunter says that the more antioxidants, the better for antiaging and health. The strongest antioxidant is melatonin, which is not meant to make you sleep, so don't take it *every* night. The dosage depends on your age. Dr. Hunter prescribes the following dosages, which should be taken every *other* night:

   - Ages 21–31: 1 mg
   - Ages 32–42: 3 mg
   - Ages 42–52: 4 mg
   - Ages 52 and older: 5 mg

   Dr. Hunter says that if you start having vivid dreams, decrease by one pill nightly until they stop. Your body knows and will tell you the perfect dosage.

   CoQ10 is an essential cofactor every time any muscle in your body contracts—think your heart muscle, too! CoQ10 is very useful for helping to treat congestive heart failure. The cholesterol-lowering drugs destroy CoQ10, which is why people get muscle aches and pains when they take them. CoQ10 also gives you energy, protects the brain, and works with the other antioxidants to make them last longer.

According to Dr. Hunter, everyone should take alpha-lipoic acid because it regenerates other antioxidants, so they last longer and you get more antiaging bang for your buck! It considerably slows down the ticking of the clock. It also helps clean your liver, detoxifies heavy metals, and lowers your blood sugar. It is great for anyone struggling with blood sugar levels, and it burns fat in higher dosages. Always take it with food. Dr. Hunter prescribes the following dosages, based on your age;

- Ages 21–35: 250 mg two times per day
- Older than 35: 600 mg per day

3. **Milk thistle:** Use this to cleanse the liver. Everyone should take this to protect the liver, which is being constantly assaulted by what we eat and breathe, in particular drugs, alcohol, chemicals, and pollution. Dr. Hunter prescribes 250 mg per day.

4. **Extra B vitamins:** Dr. Hunter prefers a "stress" dose with extra folate, because we all rush around and we're stressed both emotionally and physically. B vitamins should always be taken with food. They are water soluble, so they do make your urine yellow, but this means that they've been absorbed. B vitamins are great for the skin, hair, and nails, and decrease inflammation in the body. B vitamins, as is true for virtually all vitamins, are better taken in capsule form rather than a hard pill, because hard pills risk not getting digested or absorbed.

5. **A good-quality fish-oil supplement:** Most people don't take nearly enough. Dr. Hunter prescribes:

- Ages 21–35: At least 1,000 mg per day total of EPA and DHA
- Ages 35 and older: 2,000–3,000 mg per day

You need to make sure that your fish oils are molecularly distilled, which means they have been screened and have had any pollution removed. I highly recommend the company Nordic Naturals (www.nordicnaturals.com). This eco-responsible company carries an enormous range of top-quality fish oils and has a strong commitment to sustainable practices.

ENZYMES

Digestive enzymes are made by our bodies and are found in raw foods. They are essential for the process of digestion because they break the major nutrients in food down to molecules that are small enough to be absorbed.

There are many reasons why we don't get enough enzymes from our food. Sterile land, high-temperature preparation, and pasteurization inhibit and destroy these naturally occurring enzymes. As we age, our pancreas produces less digestive enzymes, owing to stress, genetics, and just plain old aging. Add to this the fact that most of us eat predominantly cooked foods, it's no wonder that many people over the age of forty experience regular gas, bloating, and indigestion—symptoms of bad digestion. Rather than reaching for an antacid, some of which contain the nerve toxin aluminum, try taking a good digestive enzyme. It must contain HCL (hydrochloric acid) or betaine as well as lipases, proteases, amylase, papain, bromelain, and cellulases to be useful. Dr. Hunter recommends that anyone over the age of forty take one or two digestive enzyme caplets with every meal. Dr. Hunter recommends Super Enzymes by NOW Foods (www.nowfoods.com).

PROBIOTICS

Probiotic supplements can be useful in controlling inflammatory diseases, treating and preventing allergic diseases, preventing cancer, and stimulating the immune system. A great way of making sure you have the right balance of good and bad bacteria is to eat kefir or yogurt. I've included these two foods in your eating plans to make sure you get daily probiotics. Probiotics are the same as live cultures, and the following brands of kefir and yogurt contain them: Straus Family Farm, Stonyfield Farm, Fage, and Organic Valley. Keep in mind that these yogurts have *very* low doses of probiotics, so don't rely on them to get all your probiotics. Dr. Hunter recommends taking a good probiotic supplement on an empty stomach every morning. She says that it takes a month for probiotics to repopulate thoughout the entire gut and that your colon really needs them to stay healthy.

I recommend All-Flora by a great sustainable company called New Chapter (www.newchapter.com).

AS MUCH AS YOU WANT

The most inexpensive and effective way to get your antioxidants is by eating specific fruits and vegetables. An antioxidant is a molecule that is capable of slowing down or stopping the oxidation of other molecules in your body. The problem with the oxidation process is that it can produce free radicals, which can damage cells and lead to aging and disease. I recommend that you eat the following foods, which are packed with antioxidants. Eat as many as you like.

The following list shows you, in descending order, the foods that contain the highest levels of these precious antiaging molecules. I have specified when you *must* buy organic and when you should *try* to buy organic (meaning, don't avoid if the organic version isn't available).

Must buy organic means that the produce in question has been subjected to heavy pesticide spraying and therefore may contain unsafe levels of residue, particularly for children.

1. Pecans
2. Kidney beans
3. Prunes
4. Pistachios
5. Plums
6. Blueberries—*Must buy organic*
7. Raspberries—*Must buy organic*
8. Almonds
9. Apples—*Try to buy organic*
10. Broccoli
11. Watermelon
12. Potatoes (russet)
13. Carrots—*Try to buy organic*
14. Potatoes—*Try to buy organic*
15. Radishes
16. Kiwi
17. Celery—*Try to buy organic*
18. Lettuce—*Try to buy organic*
19. Sweet cherries—*Must buy organic*
20. Tomatoes—*Try to buy organic*

TOP TEN GORGEOUS SNACKS (AND WHY)

Many of us get so stuck in our eating habits that we forget about some of nature's best-kept beauty secrets. It is actually more important that you eat some of the foods listed below than it is that you plaster on expensive skin care products. It's vital to work from the inside out. I will include as many of the following Gorgeous foods as possible in the eating plan; also, try to eat them for snacks whenever you can.

1. PRUNES

Prunes are a much-overlooked snack. A moist, chewy prune is sweet and delicious. They rank as my daughter's favorite dried fruit. They have a higher antioxidant value than *any* other fruit or vegetable, so it makes perfect sense to add them to your snack cupboard as soon as possible. They are also fantastic for digestion and promoting "friendly" bacteria in your large intestine. I have added them to all your eating plans.

2. DARK CHOCOLATE

Dark chocolate has been found to have many health benefits, which, I have to say, I'm thrilled about. I used to prefer milk chocolate but, because of the health benefits, have learned to love the tasty bittersweet version. It has been shown to reduce bad cholesterol (LDL) by up to 10 percent. There is a substance in cocoa that helps the body to process nitric oxide, a chemical that is critical for healthy blood flow and blood pressure. The flavonols in cocoa prevent fatlike substances from clotting your arteries, and they have potent antioxidant properties. As if this weren't enough, dark chocolate contains serotonin, so it's a natural antidepressant. Before you go crazy buying boxes of it, make sure that the chocolate you like has the following qualities:

- Contains 70 percent cocoa or more
- Is made from cocoa butter rather than fats such as palm and coconut oil
- Is made without the use of hydrogenated or partially hydrogenated oils
- Is as dark as possible; the darker the better, because the deep color denotes more flavonoids
- Is organic, if possible, to avoid any pesticide residue
- Is fair-trade chocolate, meaning that the producers and pickers get treated fairly, and you lower your eco-impact

www.theochocolate.com
www.sjaaks.com

www.marciesweets.com

www.dagoba.com

Trader Joe's also has a great selection of organic dark chocolate.

3. FIGS

Figs are a great choice, because they contain a mega-amount of calcium, which most women need more of. They are full of fiber, which is great when trying to manage your weight, since it helps to keep your blood sugar at a consistent level. Fiber also is a natural laxative, which holds on to water and helps move waste quickly through your intestines. Fiber also makes you feel full, providing bulk without the added calories. Figs are also a fantastic source of potassium, which helps control your blood pressure. Their blood-cleansing properties also make for clear and vibrant skin.

4. BLACK KALAMATA OLIVES

These tiny fruits are absolutely packed with vitamin E, which is essential for beautiful skin. They also contain squalene, which not only boosts the immune system but also softens and smooths the skin—it is actually found in many beauty products. As if this weren't enough, olives contain polyphenols and flavonoids, which are powerful anti-oxidants. No wonder so many Greek and Italian women have enviably gorgeous skin!

5. CUCUMBER

A cucumber a day keeps the dermatologist away! Seriously—this salad staple has outstanding beautifying properties: Cucumbers minimize water-retention and bloating. They are an excellent diuretic and cleanser for the kidneys, which is important because our kidneys filter out heavy metals such as mercury, copper, DDT, and arsenic from our bloodstream. If you buy them organic, don't peel them; the skin contains silicon and chlorophyll for skin luminosity. You can also slice them and place them over your eyes to reduce puffiness.

6. WALNUTS

These delicious nuts are packed with omega-3 fatty acids in the form of alpha-linolenic acid, which is essential for building cell membranes and heart health. They make for a tasty and delicious snack any time of the day.

7. ALMONDS

Almonds lower your bad cholesterol and reduce your heart disease risk, owing to the antioxidant action of their vitamin E content. They also contain high levels of magnesium, which has a calming effect on the mind and body, and potassium, which is an important electrolyte. Electrolytes trigger thirst and so help to keep you adequately hydrated. Almonds are also high in protein and fill you up quickly. They are a perfect snack.

8. RADISHES

Radishes are a fantastic weight-loss food because they are filling and yet contain very few calories. They are an excellent detoxifier and contain a lot of vitamin C and zinc, which are great for the skin. Not only that; they contain sulfurous compounds, which can protect against cancer.

9. AVOCADO

I eat one-half an avocado almost every day because I adore them. I am lucky, living here in Southern California, that they are so readily available locally. If you, too, like them, hurrah! They are so packed with antiaging antioxidants and vitamins and minerals that they are truly a superfruit. Contrary to what many people believe, they are great for a weight-loss diet because the monounsaturated fat actually speeds up your basal metabolic rate and they quickly make you feel full, so you are less likely to binge on foods that spike your blood sugar and cause weight gain.

10. DRIED APRICOTS

Try to buy brown unsulfured apricots. Sulfites are additives that preserve the apricot and keep its bright orange color. Without the additive, the apricots are darker but have a delicious caramel-like taste. Apricots are a wonderful diet food, for they contain very few calories and are a great source of fiber. They contain a high level of vitamin A, which is important for your vision. They are also full of antioxidants. You can't go wrong with a handful of these delicious fruits.

CHAPTER TWENTY-ONE

Skin Food

NONTOXIC SKIN CARE

Since more than 60 percent of what we put on our skin is absorbed and takes only fifteen minutes to reach our bloodstream, it's safe to say that skin care products should be looked upon as food: Our skin "ingests" them, and they are supposed to nourish us. Unfortunately, in many cases, the opposite is true—far from nourishing our skin, they can wreak all kinds of damage on the delicate living organism that is our skin: From skin irritation to hormonal disruption, even cancer, many of these pretty-looking lotions and potions should be treated with as much disdain as pesticide-laden food. How does your bathroom cabinet look? Have you started on the road to nontoxic skin care? You can always download my cheat sheet from www.gorgeouslygreen.com to help you know what to avoid when you're in the store.

There are also many foods that can be used directly on your skin for ultimate gorgeousness.

ECOLICIOUS SKIN CARE RECIPES

The following recipes contain simple and basic kitchen foods. Ask a girlfriend over for a spa night, prepare her a delicious dinner from the recipe section, and choose a face and hair mask from the recipes below. You will have a lot of fun and it will cost you next to nothing.

The following face masks are deliciously messy, so have loads of towels or a tarp on hand. Be prepared to wash your hair afterward, since it'll be covered with delicious, goopy food.

BANANARAMA NOURISHING FACE MASK

This is a rich and nourishing face mask for dry skin.

- **1 egg yolk**
- **1 ripe banana**
- **2 tsp sesame oil**

Mash all the ingredients into a paste. Before you apply to your face, set a timer for ten minutes, then pack it on! Quickly lie down with a towel under your head. Close your eyes and breathe deeply. Once the timer goes off, wash off with warm water and moisturize with a few drops of sesame oil.

HONEY AND AVOCADO MASK
FOR TIRED-LOOKING SKIN

If your skin is in need of a pick-me-up, this is the mask you need.

- **1 ripe avocado**
- **1 tsp clear honey**
- **1 tsp plain yogurt**
- **A few drops of lemon juice**
- **A few drops of aloe vera gel**

Mash all the ingredients together and leave in the fridge for an hour. When you are ready, set your timer for ten minutes, apply the mask, and lie down with a towel under your head. Wash off with warm water, pat dry, and then apply a few generous drops of pure aloe vera gel all over your face to tighten and freshen skin before applying your moisturizer.

CITRUS TONING MASK

This is a gentle exfoliating and refreshing mask that is excellent to do at least once a week. It is rich in alpha hydroxy acids, which help to gently remove the dead skin cells, leaving your skin looking shiny and new.

1 grapefruit
1 tsp lemon juice
1 cup plain yogurt
½ cup aloe vera juice

Peel the grapefruit and divide the fruit into segments. Remove the seeds and pith (white skin around each segment), place in a blender with the yogurt and lemon juice, and blend until smooth. Transfer to a small bowl and leave in the fridge for one hour. When you are ready, set your timer for ten minutes, apply your mask, and lie with a towel under your head. Wash off with warm water and pat your skin dry. Soak a cotton pad in the aloe vera juice and wipe gently over your entire face and neck.

BANANA AND COCONUT HAIR AND SCALP TREATMENT

I love this treatment—it is so messy and so fun!

1 ripe banana
2 tsp virgin coconut oil
1 cup apple cider vinegar

Simply mash the banana with the oil and apply to shampooed hair. Shove all of your hair into a shower cap (sticky, I know!) and go watch TV or read a book for thirty minutes. When you are done, shampoo again and then rinse your hair with a cup of apple cider vinegar, which is excellent for restoring the pH balance of your scalp and lays the cuticle of your hair flat. The vinegar, although acidic, is fine for color-treated hair.

ALMOND AND YOGURT QUICK HAIR SHINE

A few drops of sweet almond oil
1 cup plain yogurt

If you want to give your hair a bit more luster, rub sweet almond oil into your hair and scalp. Leave it in for a couple of hours and then rub in the yogurt. Leave for another thirty minutes before shampooing with a gentle shampoo. Try to find a shampoo that doesn't contain sodium lauryl sulphate (SLS), for this can be very harsh on your hair and scalp. Also look for a paraben-free shampoo; parabens are hormone disruptors.

Light Green

Go through your skin care products if you haven't already, with the cheat sheet in one hand, and look for the worst offenders. Add two new organic or nontoxic items to your skin care regimen this week—start with things that cover the largest area of your body, like shampoo or body lotion.

Bright Green

You have probably purged your cabinet already and replaced many of your toxic products, so this week, why not save some money, have some fun, and try out one of the ecolicious masks.

Deep Green

I know that you're a fully nontoxic, organic girl, so I throw you the challenge of making an ecolicious face *and* hair treatment this week. You won't believe how messy, fun, and effective they are!

SECTION SEVEN

Organic Girl

CHAPTER TWENTY-TWO

The Truth About Organic Food

Do you really need to fork out the extra dollars for organic food? In an ideal world, I would buy everything organic, just to make sure that my food contains the optimal amount of nutrients and no pesticide residue. I also like to lessen my eco-impact by supporting farmers who take care of our environment. However, I don't have time to schlep around the countryside looking for organic farms; moreover, organic food doesn't always work for my budget. I simply make a list of the most important foods that I need to buy organic and go from there.

Here's a list of the top ten foods to buy organic. Many of them are especially important if you have children:

1. BABY FOOD

A baby's body is extremely vulnerable to the effects of toxins because of its size and because it's growing so rapidly. Baby food is also a very concentrated form of produce, so the pesticide residue could be greater. Organic baby food in jars has become widely available at most grocery chains; if you make your own, choose organic fruits and veggies.

2. MEAT: BEEF AND CHICKEN

Most beef in this country is produced in concentrated animal feed operations (CAFOs), which might just as well be called concentration camps. The animals are basically made to eat what they shouldn't really be eating: In the case of cows, this is corn, when their systems were designed to eat grass. Their living conditions are crowded to the point that they can barely move, and the feed is laced with antibiotics, hormones, and offal to fatten them up at an abnormal speed. These horrific and un-natural living conditions give rise to frequent outbreaks of disease and so they are pumped full of even more drugs. What ends up in your grocery store is a piece of this hormone-ridden beef, which has probably been fattened with genetically modified corn; it has been packed onto a polystyrene tray in a modified-atmosphere packaging plant (low levels of oxygen) and covered with the kind of plastic that leaches. Oh—one more thing: The meat has likely been injected with a saline solution to make it appear juicier and red, as opposed to the brown color that it would be after days on a shelf.

So now you get the picture—conventionally raised beef is healthy for neither you nor the environment and is extremely cruel to animals. However, if you pick out meat that is "Certified Organic," at least you can be sure that you are avoiding the hormones and antibiotics. If the treatment of the animals is important to you, make sure you look for the "Certified Humane" label.

Chickens have an equally horrendous fate: In their concentration camps, they are fed and reared in such as way as to grow to be full-size chickens in a matter of days instead of months. Their breasts become so enormous that they cannot move at all, or their legs break under their weight, and their beaks are clipped off so that in their appalling frustration, they don't peck each other to death. Their legs and bodies are often covered in ammonia burns from having to wade around in their own waste. Their abnormally rapid breast growth also gives rise to tough, spongy meat, so it has to be pumped with saline water and chemicals. So that's what you are likely dealing with when you virtuously prepare your lightly grilled, boneless, skinless chicken breast and salad! If you have ever tasted a chicken that has been pecking around a farmyard (my grandmother kept chickens), it is a different story: much smaller and tasty, naturally juicy meat. Needless to say, if you still want to eat chicken, make sure it's "Certified Organic" and "Free Range," which means it must have *some* outside access and it must be fed on an entirely organic diet without hormones or antibiotics. Even better, go and find a farm online or near you so you can actually check out the conditions—I personally don't fancy eating a chicken that has suffered for its entire life. It just doesn't feel right. So next time you go to the grocery store, think care-fully before you reach for those super-size chicken breasts and consider for a moment exactly how they came to be so ridiculously enormous.

3. DAIRY PRODUCTS AND EGGS

This might be the most important item for you to change if you and your family consume a lot of dairy. You will see some dairy products labeled "organic" and some labeled "rBGH-free." The latter refers to dairies that have agreed not to use the bovine growth hormone, which has been banned in Japan and Europe. The organic label refers to dairies that have to feed the cows organic grain, use no growth hormones or antibiotics, and give the cow access to outside pasture. I choose organic milk because my young daughter consumes a lot of dairy and I don't want her to be getting a dose of antibiotics with her cereal. "Certified Organic" is the only label that has third-party verification.

Organic eggs are great because the certification means that the chicken hasn't touched a grain that isn't organic. However, they can be a lot more expensive. If you are eating eggs by themselves, the taste of organic is so much better. If you are using them for baking or cooking recipes, you may want to go for conventional to save money. Avoid dried or liquid egg products, which might contain hydrogenated fats, artificial flavor and color, preservatives, sugar, fructose, corn syrup, or soy protein.

4. RICE AND RICE CEREAL

Conventional rice crops rely on heavy pesticide usage. The groundwater around most rice paddies in both California and Asia has been found to be heavily contaminated. Buy organic brown rice in bulk when you can; it's less expensive. Also make sure that any baby's rice cereal, often their first food, is organic.

5. GRAINS: WHEAT, CORN, AND OATS

Pesticide residue has been found in many leading brands of breakfast cereal. Processed foods made with corn (corn chips, tortillas, popcorn, and corn bread) are among the top foods that are likely to expose children to unsafe doses of organophosphate residue.

6. TOMATO KETCHUP

Since more than 75 percent of the tomatoes grown in the United States are used for processed foods, including tomato ketchup, it makes sense to make sure the tomatoes are organic. Tests have found that organic brands contain more than 50 percent more antioxidants, and it's a great way to get these valuable nutrients into kids.

7. PEANUT BUTTER

Most peanut farms in the United States use conventional farming practices, including the use of fungicide to keep the mold at bay. Since these fungicide and pesticide residues can mount up when our kids eat peanut butter almost every day, it makes sense to switch to the organic kind. Organic peanut butter is also less likely to contain additives like high-fructose corn syrup.

8. POTATOES

As potatoes are a daily staple for many of us, I have included them on this list. Conventionally farmed potatoes have been discovered to contain more pesticides than any other vegetable, even after being peeled and washed. In 2006, the USDA conducted a study in which they found that, after being washed and peeled, 81 percent of potatoes still contained pesticides.

9. APPLES

Apple juice, applesauce, and whole, crunchy apples should be organic whenever possible. Apples are one of the top pesticide-heavy fruit crops, so if you and your family eat a lot of them, switch to organic.

10. STRAWBERRIES

Strawberries are the most heavily contaminated produce item in the United States. I have included them on this list since conventionally grown strawberries are available year-round and should be avoided at all costs.

PRODUCE

Whether you can get them organic or not, eat mounds of fresh fruits and veggies. You don't need to buy *everything* organic, and if you can find only a few wilted old vegetables in the store, it's probably best to buy conventional. Remember that a fruit or vegetable's nutrient content is directly related to how long it's been on the shelf. The clock starts ticking the moment the fruit has been picked, and the closer you are to that moment, the more you'll get what nature intended.

Here's a short list of the produce items that I recommend you buy organic. They are listed in descending order of importance:

1. Strawberries
2. Peaches
3. Nectarines
4. Pears
5. Apples
6. Celery
7. Sweet bell peppers
8. Potatoes
9. Spinach
10. Lettuce

Here is a longer list of the produce items that you *don't* need to buy organic:

1. Asparagus
2. Avocados
3. Bananas
4. Broccoli
5. Cauliflower
6. Sweet corn
7. Kiwi
8. Mango
9. Onions
10. Papayas
11. Pineapples
12. Sweet peas
13. Eggplant
14. Cabbage

PESTIDICES ASIDE

Aside from pesticides, what are the other reasons we should buy organic food? Pesticide residue isn't the only thing to worry about with conventionally produced food. When we look into what's behind the organic label, we can begin to understand the true nature of conventional farming.

To be "Certified Organic" with the green-and-white USDA label, a food:

- Must be grown without pesticides, herbicides, and nitrogen fertilizers—all of which are made from fossil fuels
- Must not use any genetically modified seeds
- Must not use sewage sludge
- Must not use radiation

Let's look into each of these aspects of organic farming in a little more detail. I had no idea that my nonorganic food was sometimes steeped in animal poop, blasted with radioactive rays, and contained genetically modified ingredients. What does all this mean, and although all these things sound bad, are they really going to affect my health? Read on and make your own informed decisions from now on.

PESTICIDES, HERBICIDES, AND CHEMICAL FERTILIZERS

Pesticides, herbicides, and fertilizers are known as "inputs" in the agricultural industry. They are made from fossil fuels, so they will become more expensive as oil prices rise. These inputs starting being used after World War II, when the munitions factories that developed nitrogen-based chemicals for warfare had to find something new to do with them. They discovered that they made crops grow really fast, but what they didn't realize was that these chemicals not only destroy the natural eco-balance of the soil, leaving it useless after a few growing seasons, but also run off or leach into the planet's water systems, creating widespread pollution—and that's just the start of it. These chemicals allowed farmers to produce massive monocrops (meaning that a farmer will grow just one crop instead of four or five) and thus initially bolstered food production, but these "inputs" quickly destroy the fertility of the soil so that more and more chemicals have to be added to keep up with demand. Also factor in the fact that the damage they have caused to ecosystems, animals, and yes, humans, is now almost irreversible. Because these chemicals deplete the soil so badly, more land has to be used up as farmers move on. The old method of crop rotation was so much more beneficial for the environment and fruitful. In an ideal world, it would be wonderful to go back to the small-scale organic farming of yesteryear. However, with more than 6 billion people on the planet now (estimated to grow to more than nine billion by 2030), we've got a bit of a challenge ahead of us. I think organic farming is the way to go, because we need to restore biodiversity and soil health, and contrary to what many people believe, organic farming can eventually produce equal if not higher yields than conventional farming.

Organic farming produces foods that are far superior nutritionally. In numerous scientific tests, organically grown produce has been found to contain much higher levels of the very vitamins and minerals we need to keep us disease free and gorgeous. Many studies have concluded that organic foods contain substantially higher levels of flavonoids (antioxidants), vitamin C, iron, magnesium, and phosphorus—all hugely important in staying young and healthy. The more we shop for organic food, the more demand we create. So vote with your dollars, and the food industry will get the message loud and clear: We demand healthy food for ourselves, our children, and the planet, and we'll accept nothing less!

Pesticides are a scarier story: If they can destroy the nervous system of an insect, they can do the same to us. They have been used so liberally over the past thirty years that superbugs are now developing that are resistant to many of these chemicals, so farmers just have to spray more and more pesticide in the hope that the bugs will go away—they won't! It's the same with herbicides. Farmers are now finding superweeds (think Little Shop of Horrors). Weeds are very crafty; they want to strangle and deplete healthy plants with a vengeance and so they've found a way around these herbicides, resulting in heavier spraying. Did you know that the average plant crop gets ten separate applications of pesticide before it even reaches the storage unit? Many of the everyday foods we pick on account of their health benefits are, ironically, covered in a pesticide residue that doesn't wash off under the kitchen faucet.

It's worth noting that organic food isn't always the only way to go: There are many farmers in the United States who are producing sustainable food that doesn't harm the environment, yet they cannot get the USDA organic seal because they may still use a little herbicide or nitrogen fertilizer. These farmers are often the middle-size farmers who are trying to cater to the enormous demand for sustainable food, which the small "alternative farmers" cannot. Many of them have developed incredibly innovative, eco-friendly farming methods, yet that little bit of fertilizer takes them out of the picture as far as the organic label is concerned. You will also find small-scale farmers at your farmer's market, who cannot afford to get the organic seal (pretty costly), so they cannot tell you that their wares are organic—though you will find, if you ask, that many of them do not use pesticides or herbicides. We need to get off the buzzword bandwagon and make informed choices based on the answers we get. When you are at a farmer's market, ask the vendors about their growing methods. The most important thing that you need to check is that they don't spray pesticides. You can even ask where their farm is and mention that you would love to visit them soon.

GMO FOODS

If you lived in Europe, you would know a lot more about genetically modified food because the public is up in arms about it. They think they have a right to know if their food has been genetically modified, and they've forced government to put strict labeling regulations into place. I agree with them, and here's why.

First off—what are genetically modified foods? They are plants or seeds that have had their genetic makeup altered so that they become more efficient. They are "designer" plants that either grow more quickly or are more disease resistant or produce vegetables that are absolutely uniform in shape or size or have a longer shelf life, and so on. That doesn't sound so bad until you learn about the process that makes this possible. Inserting a foreign gene into a plant is no easy task—it's a hit-or-miss operation. As Andrew Kimbrell says in his excellent book *Your Right to Know,* "Some corporate scientists call genetic engineering a precise technology; the truth is it's anything but exact. Every time they insert a novel gene into a plant cell, the gene ends up in a random location in the plant's genome. As a result, each new gene amounts to a game of food-safety roulette, leaving companies hoping that the new gene, its cassette and whatever location it arrived in, will not destabilize a new food and make it toxic."

Many genetically modified seed engineers employ the Terminator Technology, which is designed to genetically switch off a plant's ability to germinate a second time. This requires farmers to buy new seeds every year and therefore is crippling many farmers in developing nations.

You may wonder why the FDA and our government haven't taken the whole GMO industry to task, but sadly there is a lot of money to be made and lobbyists are doing their thing, so in the United States, these health threats have been largely ignored. Right now, there is no mandatory testing for the short- and long-term toxicity of GMO foods. Since they have only been around since the 1990s, the possibility of dangerous long-term effects really scares me. I'm not a risk taker when it comes to health, so I want to stay away from GMO foods whenever I can.

It's a little alarming to discover that more than 60 percent of processed foods in our grocery stores contain GMO ingredients. If you are buying conventionally produced food, know that the genetic engineering can lower the nutritional content of the food. A study by Dr. Marc Lappé published in the *Journal of Medicinal Food* found that concentrations of beneficial phytoestrogen compounds, which protect against heart disease and cancer, were lower in genetically modified soybeans than in traditional strains.

Many of these GMO crops are engineered to be herbicide resistant, which means that farmers can spray as much herbicide as they want without damaging the crop. This could triple the amount of toxic herbicides currently used in agriculture.

People with allergies can be seriously harmed by exposure to foreign proteins that, with genetic modification, are spliced into common foods. The FDA doesn't require premarket testing to determine if new allergens or toxins are present in GMO foods. We should be particularly careful on behalf of babies and small children, because their immune systems are not fully developed and diseases later in life can be traced back to early childhood diet. One wonders why childhood asthma has doubled since the eighties, and autism and attention deficit disorder are now common occurrences.

An easy way to avoid most GMO foods is to buy only products with the USDA organic seal on them. The rules that earn a company this seal prohibit the use of GMO plants or ingredients—a very good reason to buy organic.

The most frightening thing about genetically modified seeds is that they could threaten our food security. The Prince of Wales has spoken out against the global GMO industry, saying that the development of these crops could be the "world's worst environmental disaster." He goes on to say "that it would be the absolute destruction of everything and the classic way of ensuring there is no food in the future."

IRRADIATION

This is when your food is zapped to ostensibly remove any bacteria that may be lurking—great in theory, as many of these practices seem. However, a rather shady picture emerges when you scratch beneath the surface. First off, the practice of irradiation masks the filthy and unsanitary conditions of most factory farms, where disease and bacteria are prevalent. In an ideal world, these factories would have to clean up their acts rather than relying on having their meat shot through with X-rays (more powerful than anything a human could withstand) and gamma rays.

These rays break apart bacteria and insects that may be hidden in the food, but they create by-products, which according to the Center for Food Safety include a variety of mutagens—substances that can cause gene mutations, polyploidy (an abnormal condition in which cells contain more than two sets of chromosomes), chromosome aberrations (often associated with cancerous cells), and dominant lethal mutations (a change in a cell that prevents it from reproducing) in human cells. Making matters worse, many mutagens are also carcinogens. Irradiation can also destroy the vitamin content of the food.

There is currently a law that requires producers to label the product as "Treated by Irradiation," though the FDA, pressured by industry, may change this label to something that serves to fool consumers like you and me—the label will read "Electronically Pasteurized" or "Cold Pasteurized," which sounds a lot better, but its no different.

SEWAGE SLUDGE

When you flush your toilet or rinse off a paintbrush in your kitchen, you may be unknowingly contributing to the stew of chemicals that are used to fertilize the food that ends up on your table. The government disposes of unwanted by-products from municipal wastewater treatment plants by selling it off to farmers as sewage sludge for fertilizing their crops.

This is almost the worst of the bunch as far as I'm concerned. Sewage sludge is what the name suggests. In the industry, they call it biosolids, which doesn't sound so disgusting, but it's still recycled human poop.

Many say that there's nothing wrong with this kind of fertilizer and that it's better it not go to waste. However, the problem lies in the fact that it's not just poop and pee, it's a plethora of toxic substances, too. Anything that goes down our drain ends up in this sewage sludge: paint thinner, drugs, toxic skin care products, and more. Many of these compounds cannot and do not break down and miraculously disappear in the treatment plant—no, sir! They end up fertilizing your conventionally grown strawberries, green beans, and everything else you eat to try to stay healthy. Residents living near some of the thousands of fields that apply sewage sludge have become very sick, and there have even been deaths as a direct result of bacterial poisoning.

STAYING INFORMED

So there you have it. Conventionally produced food employs all of the above and gets a food on your plate that may look good with its shiny, waxed skin and uniform shape, but honestly you'd be so much better off with a crooked green bean or a misshapen tomato that actually was grown as nature intended it to be.

Keep in mind that it's not always black and white, especially where small- and middle-size farmers are concerned. Don't write a producer off because he or she is not "Certified Organic." There may be plenty of great farms that may apply a little herbicide or pesticide but that eschew most of the above practices. Now that you are more informed, if you find a farmer or farm you like, you can ask exactly how they produce their food.

Stay as informed as you can about organic food by visiting www.organic consumers.org and food safety at www.foodandwaterwatch.com.

LOCAVORE?

A big deal has been made about the importance of buying local food over the last few years, but what's all the fuss about? If I want to eat bananas and I live in England, local just isn't going to work. Anyway, what's wrong with providing indigenous or third-world communities with a local economy—we've all got to make a living! Whether or not you agree with globalization or free trade between countries, being Gorgeously Green is all about awareness, and it's vital to scrutinize every item you pick up at the store. Avoiding globalization and eschewing food from the other side of the globe is an extremely hard thing to do for most of us. If you like vanilla, cinnamon, spices, pepper, coffee, tea, and so on, you'd be hard-pressed to find any of these items produced locally. But, given the fact that each meal we eat travels an average of

12,000 miles to get from the farm to our kitchen, we might want to look at the implications of this elongated travel time.

Fruits and vegetables are obviously at their absolute best when they are just plucked off the plant or tree—at that moment, they are brimming with every nutrient and enzyme that nature intended. They are "living" foods that make you feel energized and alive. As these veggies are packed into crates, this goodness begins to diminish, and as each hour ticks by, more and more nutrients are lost. Add to this the numerous methods used to extend shelf life (modified-atmosphere packaging, gassing, and spraying), and the nutrients have a hard time staying alive at all—and we haven't even gotten to the truck or airplane yet! These food miles will not provide you with the healthiest foods, and if you want to lessen your eco-impact, you may want to find out where your apples or peaches were grown, as you don't want to factor too much fossil fuel into the equation.

All in all, it makes the most sense to keep scrutinizing the labels and start making informed decisions. I choose not to buy green beans that come from Africa, or apples that come from New Zealand, because they've had to travel too far. Admittedly, many of my daily staples, from coffee to coconut oil, come from thousands of miles away, but being Bright Green, I'm not willing to part with them yet. I'm always on the lookout to buy local whenever I can, and obviously the ideal place for that is the farmer's market. I try to buy 90 percent of my produce from these local vendors, and whatever else I can get from there—pastries, cheese, olive oil, and even jewlry! Sometimes I have to travel a bit to get to this fantastic farmer's market that has the best herbed goat cheese I have ever tasted, grass-fed bison, which is superb, and a family bakery whose loaves I treasure (actually hide from my family) until the last crumb has disappeared.

Another part of the jigsaw of eco-friendly eating is to make sure that you try to eat seasonal produce. This really goes hand in hand with the local thing, in that seasonal foods are much more nutritious because they have not been forced to grow out of season. We have now become so used to eating summer fruits and vegetables all year round that it is a bit of a shock if you decide to buy only what's in season. I can't help feeling a bit cheated at my farmer's market in the winter, looking around and not seeing any red bell peppers or berries—hmmm—what on earth am I going to do with a bunch of ugly-looking root vegetables? It's especially tough if I've got a particular dish or recipe that I'm craving. It serves me well to remember that when I was growing up in England, we simply didn't have a choice, for we ate primarily what came out of the garden. The thrill of the first tomatoes and raspberries in the summer is a memory I will always treasure. I can actually taste those warm, puffy berries that we'd pluck straight from the bush and cram into our mouths. We ate and ate them every which way, with sugar, clotted cream, pastries, pies, and mousses until the season was over and we moved on to the gooseberries or pears. The seasons were marked by our food, but things still traveled, even back then: I remember when December came around and we'd get oranges from faraway, exotic-sounding places, which were so much of a treat that Santa would often stuff one down our stocking, along with a walnut. If I put a piece of fruit in Lola's stocking now, she'd think that good old Santa had totally lost the plot. We've become too blasé and bored with our food. This will change over the next few years, primarily because of oil prices—we simply will not be able to afford food that has had to travel too far, so one of the few upsides of peak oil prices is that we may learn to treasure seasonal food once again.

FLEXITARIAN

I consider myself to be a "flexitarian" in that I eat mostly vegetables and fruit, a little meat and fish, and everything that is delicious in moderation! I am also extremely flexible, because I never want my diet to be restrictive. I adore traveling and sampling the culinary delights of different world cuisines and cultures. I'll give almost everything a try *once*, and in the case of chicken feet and pig's trotter, *never* again! I don't want to be a party pooper or one of those incredibly annoying guests who send their hosts into a spin, trying to accommodate them. When I'm invited to a party, being the Green Girl that I am, I'm always asked what I do and don't eat, and honestly, it gives me so much pleasure to say "I eat everything!" If I'm faced with a plastic-looking, nitrate-laden hot dog, I'll politely take a minuscule bite, for I know it's not going to kill me, and then I help myself to a gargantuan portion of coleslaw or sweet corn. If I positively know that I'm going to be facing mounds of cheap, drug-infused meat, I sometimes suggest that I'd love to bring some special meat, fish, or veggie burgers along for everyone to try. The key is to turn people on, not off.

CHAPTER TWENTY-THREE

The Pledge

The only way we can be absolutely assured of success in making an important change is when we make a pact or a promise with ourselves *and* someone else. Since the Gorgeously Green Diet is all about lessening your eco-impact and improving your health, I have created a six-step pledge to help you to define your goals and stick to them.

In my experience, whenever I have had to let go of a bad habit or learn something new, I have had to make it public—it's the only way I will stick to it in moments of weakness. The other day, I rushed into the grocery store to buy some items for Lola's lunch box. In a moment of weakness or laziness, I grabbed a bunch of "convenience" foods that I knew would save time and energy: individually wrapped portions of carrots and ranch dressing, juice boxes, and individually wrapped slices of string cheese. As I waited impatiently in the checkout line, I felt really guilty, realizing with horror that I had told virtually all of my girlfriends that I *never* buy individually wrapped portions anymore because of all the unnecessary packaging, the manufacture and disposal of which pollutes the environment. What if one of these women spotted me, red-handed, stuffing these items into—oh, no! I had also forgotten my reusable bags! In a total panic, I ditched the basket, went back to my car for the bags, and started the whole shopping venture again. If I hadn't boasted to everyone about how Green I was, I probably would have let it go. Going public, like I did, with your new eco-friendly intentions is definitely the way to go.

TAKE THE GORGEOUSLY GREEN DIET *PLEDGE*

Read through the following six steps and then sign the pledge at the bottom of the page. Also log onto www.gorgeouslygreen.com and click on "Lean & Green Pledge" to make your pledge public on our Gorgeously Green Diet message board. Becoming part of this community will also connect you with other women who have taken the pledge. You can share ideas, tips, and insights as you go along.

1. I commit to cutting my beef and chicken consumption down by 25–50 percent. I will prepare at least three meat-free meals a week. Meat production has a very heavy eco-impact.
2. I commit to buying organic, seasonal, and locally produced food whenever possible. I vote with my dollars and want to support sustainable producers.
3. I commit to cooking at least three meals a week at home so that I can save money, my health, and the planet.
4. I commit to reducing my food waste by 50 percent by sticking to my eating plan and my shopping list and by using my leftovers.
5. I commit to growing something edible (even an herb will do!).
6. I commit to recycling my paper, plastic, glass, and cans, and to buying recycled paper products (paper towels, napkins, and toilet paper) to preserve more trees.

I, _____, pledge to take the six Gorgeously Green steps and to practice them for the next thirty days.

CHAPTER TWENTY-FOUR

Being the Change

You can make a difference before it's too late. I have heard so many stories from individuals and families who have jumped on the Green bandwagon only after a cancer scare. A scary health diagnosis will spur even the most cynical of us into doing everything within our power to rid our homes and our planet of toxins and to try to ensure an ongoing supply of clean food, soil, and water. I urge you to make the changes now and always to err on the side of caution.

Melissa, a mother at my daughter's school, was one of those women who just sort of disappeared into the background. She always seemed down, drained, and literally gray. Her skin was pale, her hair was lusterless, and she never looked at anyone. I often wondered about her and secretly thought that if she pulled herself together and at least got her hair sorted out, she might feel better. However, I didn't get to hear her story until a summer field trip. We found ourselves squashed together at a picnic table and she started telling me that she was interested in the Green initiatives that I was starting to bring into the school. She surprisingly seemed really passionate about eco-issues and came alive as she told me the changes she would like to see on the campus, too. We ended up chatting for an hour or so and she told me her story.

Up until a few years back, she had been a "regular girl" who never gave the environment a second thought. She said she had been living "unconsciously." One day, she noticed her yardman spraying the tall bushes behind her house. Apparently, they were prone to a plant disease, he thought, and so he was going to give them a good spray to make sure. She stood chatting with him while he sprayed. A few days later, she felt tired and weak and had a headache. A few weeks later she felt "fuzzy" and confused and started forgetting things. When her arms started to tremble occasionally and her legs felt like they were going to give way under her, she went to the doctor. After months of visiting all kinds of specialists and getting worse, she was diagnosed with multiple sclerosis (MS), an often crippling and degenerative disease. Wow, now it made sense that when I saw her walking her daughter to school, she shuffled along as though she had trouble keeping her balance.

Then, on a chance visit to a brilliant chiropractor, she received the first ray of hope. He was convinced she didn't have MS. The symptoms just didn't match, and so he asked her hundreds of questions about the last few years of her life. After a laborious process of examination and discovery, he traced her symptoms all the way back to the spraying of the bushes and absolutely knew without a doubt that she was suffering from pesticide poisoning. After months of intense therapy to rid her body of the toxins, she is on the road to recovery and suffers from none of the debilitating symptoms anymore.

This experience woke her up to the plight of the planet. If she had gotten so sick from one spraying of a pesticide, what about the people who worked around these chemicals day in and day out? What about pesticide residue on our food? And what about toxic cleaning supplies and unknown chemicals in our water? In her still fragile condition, she needed to be vigilant and cared passionately about these issues for her family. She told me that she used to be a Texas girl who thought Green was either for crunchie hippies or the hybrid-driving elite. She had clearly changed her mind.

Melissa's story is one of many that I have heard, and the common thread is that some kind of environmental pollutant was a catalyst for a big wake-up call. I think we can all wake up without having to suffer. We can realize that now is the time to put our best foot forward and try to make a difference. Everything counts. Whether you are installing a low-flow showerhead or cutting your beef consumption because it's the most water-intensive food on the planet, you are making a difference.

One of the most thrilling things about the Internet is that we can and should become activists from the comfort of our own home. If you only knew how much power you have with the click of a mouse. E-activists are changing the food landscape of America in an extraordinary way: It was an online nonprofit organization (www .foodandwaterwatch.org) that spearheaded the pressure initially put on Starbucks

Coffee to use only milk free of growth hormones. With further efforts from other online organizations, many other giant companies were forced to follow suit, and as a result, we are now able to buy rBGH-free milk in virtually every supermarket chain across the country. Another powerful example is the incredible online participation by farmers, gardeners, and concerned citizens in getting the U.S. Farm Bill changed: The Farm Bill has recently mandated federal support for organic food production and earmarked twenty million dollars for low-income seniors to shop at farmer's markets—now, that's progress, which has been largely created by e-activism.

How can you help? First off, think of some of the things that bother you about food production, then contact your local senator or representatives. If you are as concerned as I am about the fact that, right now, food containing GMO ingredients does not have to be labeled as such, let these people know that you want something to be done about it. Simply visit www.house.gov and click on "write your representative." When you type in your nine-digit zip code, you'll be told exactly who your representative is. You can also send a letter to your representatives by filling out your details. Write to these people who speak for us about any issue that bothers you.

I highly recommend becoming an e-activist by visiting www.foodandwater watch.org and clicking on "Take Action." It's a wonderfully informative Web site that will tell you everything you need to know about food and water, including the location of your nearest beef and poultry factory farm. You can also visit www.farm sanctuary.org and vote on campaigns. If you've got the stomach for it, you can browse some pretty sad photographs that will put you off feedlot meat for life.

If you're in the mood for a bit of voluntary work on an organic farm, visit www .organicvolunteers.com; and if you want to get involved in changes made to future farm bills (or to find out what on earth the Farm Bill is!), visit www.foodandwater watch.org or the National Family Farm Coalition (www.nffc.net). Commit to taking one action a week. There are so many aspects of food production that are devastating to the environment and our health. From dangerous chemicals in our drinking water to overstuffed, off-gassing landfills, you can help be the change with a simple click.

CHAPTER TWENTY-FIVE

Giving It Away

I'm a great believer in giving away something of what I am so blessed to have. I took a home-baked loaf over to a girlfriend the other day and I felt like June Cleaver gone Green—the only thing missing was a frilly apron and an updo. I also desperately try to score brownie points (or greenie points) by being the room mom at my daughter's school—it's also a great way of trying to control what is brought into the classroom. I've steered everyone away from bringing in juice boxes and a number of other additive-laden foods and drinks. The last class party was an unmitigated success. I think the other moms were a bit nervous about my Gorgeously Green guidelines—how on earth would the kids have fun without blue/pink frosting and goody bags? Surely we couldn't expect them to get by on drinking water instead of juice! The children came back for third helpings of the homemade banana bread and piled their plates high with raw carrots, celery, and snow peas. Instead of goody bags filled with candy and plastic toys, we played ridiculous games and the kids laughed until they had tears streaming down their cheeks. Lola said it was the best party *ever*. Her teacher was delighted, for she had a class of calm and happy kids to read to that afternoon. She also said that when given a choice, the kids pick homemade food over store-bought stuff every time. So if you're a goody-goody mom like me, let that be your way of giving. Take it over the top and bake the teacher a loaf of banana bread, too.

Another great way of giving is to cook something for someone who is housebound or sick. If you've ever visited a retirement home, you'll see that so much of what they are fed is low-quality pap. If you know anyone in such an establishment, get a few extra fruits and veggies at the farmer's market and bake them a treat. If anyone in my neighborhood is going through a hard time (divorce, family emergency—whatever), a group of us get together online and organize a roster of who will do dinner on which night. I remember after coming back from the hospital with baby Lola, exhausted and depressed, and I got a homemade dinner dropped off at my doorstep every night for a week—along with home-baked bread and cookies and fresh organic fruit. I'll remember to this day what each woman brought because it meant the world to me.

GREEN COMMUNITY

The most important action we can take in living an earth-friendly life is to think and act as a community. One definition of community is "a group of people with a common background or shared interests within society." By virtue of living in the same area, you have a common background, and if you can find a handful of people who are interested in living a greener way of life, you're onto a good thing. Reach out to your neighbors and invite them to take the Gorgeously Green Diet Pledge.

For years, I had a neighbor whom I never spoke to. We clearly had very little in common, other than living on the same street. One day he planted, of all things, a banana tree in the tiny space between our houses. It was disputable whether this space belonged to him or us, but as the tree grew into a wild and wonderful fruit-bearing monstrosity, who cared? He then started planting other weird-looking crops around the base of the tree—hmmmm—this chap was clearly into biodiversity and could teach me a thing or two. One day I saw him in the parking lot of our local health food store and I rushed up to him. He *sort* of recognized me as his neighbor but wondered what I wanted (people are always suspicious nowadays)—I just told him that I loved his banana tree (ha!) and was fascinated to know about what other things he was growing. This led to a half-hour conversation during which we realized that we were both urban gardeners or were at least trying to be. Since then, he has been around with lemons, artichokes, and eggs—I thought I had heard some clucking.

You will get great satisfaction from joining a CSA (community supported agriculture) or community garden. Any activity that brings people together for the common good has tremendous power and magic in it. I often fantasize about living in a little old-fashioned village somewhere. This fantasy village is surrounded by fields of organic vegetables, fruit orchards, and bleating baby lambs. The reality is that I live in the smoggy urban sprawl of Los Angeles. I *have* to drive, there isn't a field of any kind in sight, and the only glimpse of a live animal I get is either Zoom the stray cat (who's addicted to my organic milk) or Rosemary the resident compost bin rat.

I have, however, found a way of living and eating that reflects my deeper values and feels, for the most part, utterly fantastic. While I carry on dreaming, if I may, of that organic orchard that I will be skipping through one day, I pledge to practice the six Gorgeously Green Steps in my life in the hope that each day I can experience a little bit of heaven on earth.

SECTION EIGHT

Recipes

BREAKFAST

Smoothies to die for! I adore smoothies because you can pack so much goodness into one delicious shot. I recommend using whey or hemp protein powder in the six smoothie recipes that follow. Just combine all the ingredients in a blender and blend until smooth. They each make 1 serving.

For whey or hemp protein powders, see p. 45.

TROPICAL BREAKFAST SMOOTHIE

If you haven't got time for breakfast, or you're just not hungry, this will make sure you get all the good stuff and should keep you going for a few hours.

1 8-ounce glass almond milk
1 scoop whey protein powder
½ mango, papaya, or orange
½ ripe banana
1 tbsp virgin coconut oil
1 tbsp rolled oats

BERRY BREAKFAST SMOOTHIE

1 8-ounce glass almond milk
1 scoop whey or hemp protein powder
½ cup seasonal berries (use frozen organic if not in season)
1 tbsp flaxseed oil
1 tbsp rolled oats

PEANUT BUTTER GOOD-MOOD FOOD

This is my daughter's favorite!

1 8-ounce glass almond milk
1 tbsp peanut butter
2 heaping tsp cocoa powder
1 tsp raw agave syrup

CRAZY CRANBERRY SMOOTHIE

1 8-ounce glass almond milk
1 scoop whey protein powder
½ ripe banana
1 tbsp virgin coconut oil
1 tbsp pure unsweetened cranberry juice
1 tbsp dried unsweetened coconut

ALMOND ANGEL SMOOTHIE

1 8-ounce glass almond milk
1 scoop whey or hemp protein powder
1 ripe banana
2 tbsp almond butter
2 tsp agave syrup

GORGEOUSLY GREEN SMOOTHIE

1 8-ounce glass almond milk
1 scoop hemp or hemp protein powder

½ ripe banana
½ cup fresh seasonal berries (if not in season, use frozen organic)
1 tsp green superfoods powder (page 46)
1 tsp agave syrup

NUTTY GRANOLA

½ cup honey or agave syrup
¼ cup virgin coconut oil
1 tsp vanilla extract
4 cups rolled oats
½ cup raw almonds
½ cup walnut pieces
½ cup sunflower seeds
½ cup shredded unsweetened coconut
1 cup raisins
½ cup unsweetened dried cranberries or apricots cut into small pieces

Preheat the oven to 375°F.

Combine the honey/agave syrup and coconut oil in a small saucepan over low heat and warm until liquefied. Add the vanilla.

Combine the oats, almonds, walnuts, sunflower seeds, and coconut in a large bowl and add the honey mixture. Mix well to evenly coat and spread over a baking sheet.

Place in the oven and bake for 10 minutes, then stir until lightly brown and return to the oven for a further 10 minutes or until crisp and lightly browned. Remove from the oven and add the dried fruit. Allow to cool before storing in a large glass or stainless steel container for up to one month.

HOMEMADE ALMOND MILK

1 cup raw almonds
You will also need: unbleached cheesecloth
Yield: about 4 cups almond milk

Put the almonds in a glass bowl and cover with 4 cups water. Refrigerate overnight. Drain, rinse, and put in the blender with 3 cups fresh water. Blend until smooth. Strain through a cheesecloth-lined strainer into a pitcher.

To sweeten, return the almond milk to the blender and blend with 3 or 4 dates that have been soaked in water for a couple of hours, or make a delicious Gorgeously Green shake by blending with ½ banana, 1 tsp green superfoods (page 46), and 1 tsp agave syrup.

COCONUT PROTEIN PANCAKES

Everyone is crazy about my coconut pancakes. Not only are they scrumptious, but they'll keep you going until lunch because of the coconut oil and protein.

Serves 2–3
3 eggs
1 cup cottage cheese
½ cup whole-grain pancake mix
1 tbsp shredded unsweetened coconut
2 tbsp virgin coconut oil

Whisk the eggs in a large bowl and mix in the cottage cheese. Stir in the pancake mix and shredded coconut.

Heat the coconut oil in a nonstick skillet over medium-high heat. Drop the batter into the skillet (2 tablespoons per pancake) and cook until the underside is set and lightly colored and bubbles form on top, then flip and cook until set and lightly colored on the other side.

Serve with a little pure maple syrup or brown rice syrup and sliced strawberries or bananas.

ORANGE BRAN FLAX MUFFINS

This was one of the runner-up recipe winners in a recipe competition we held at www.gorgeously green.com. I love that every ingredient is extremely healthy. These are absolutely delicious, and I highly recommend making the full amount (24 muffins) and freezing half for another time.

Makes 24
1½ cups oat bran
1 cup all-purpose flour
1 cup flaxseed, ground
1 cup wheat bran
1 tbsp baking powder

½ tsp salt
2 oranges, quartered and seeded
1 cup brown sugar
1 cup buttermilk
½ cup canola oil or coconut oil
2 eggs
1 tsp baking soda
1½ cups golden raisins (optional)

Preheat the oven to 375°F.

Line two 12-cup muffin pans with paper liners or coat the pans with cooking spray. In a large bowl, combine the oat bran, flour, flaxseed, wheat bran, baking powder, and salt. Set aside.

In a blender or food processor, combine the oranges, brown sugar, buttermilk, oil, eggs, and baking soda. Blend well.

Pour the orange mixture into the dry ingredients. Mix until well blended. Then stir in the raisins.

Divide the batter evenly among the muffin cups. Bake for 18 to 20 minutes, or until a toothpick inserted in the center comes out clean. Cool in the pans for 5 minutes before removing to a cooling rack.

COCONUT, WALNUT, AND BANANA MUFFINS

These are amazingly healthy, filling, and delicious. I made them with coconut flour because it's so nutritious. You can easily find coconut flour at a good health store or at www.tropicaltraditions.com, or you can substitute the coconut flour with whole-wheat flour. If you use the coconut flour, these muffins have a very different consistency from regular muffins. The mixture will be thicker and the finished muffin is denser and more crumbly, but so good! They are spectacular if served warm with a little butter or ghee, and they'll store in an airtight container for a week.

Makes 12 muffins
1 cup organic coconut flour
1 tsp aluminum-free baking powder
3 tbsp shredded unsweetened coconut
½ cup walnut pieces
2 bananas, mashed

6 eggs

2 tbsp butter, melted

3 tbsp virgin coconut oil

1/2 cup milk

3 tbsp honey

1 tsp vanilla extract

1/4 tsp salt

Preheat the oven to 350°F. Liberally grease a 12-cup muffin pan.

Combine the coconut flour and baking powder in a large bowl. Add the shredded coconut and walnut pieces. In a food processor, process the remaining ingredients until smooth, then carefully fold into the flour mixture. Spoon the mixture into the muffin pan and bake for 20 minutes or until they are firm to the touch and lightly browned. Remove and cool on a wire rack. Store in an airtight container for up to a week.

LUNCH

WALDORF SALAD

This is a light and healthy version of the classic Waldorf. A perfect winter salad.

Serves 4

1/2 cup plain Greek yogurt or sour cream

1/2 cup Spectrum canola mayonnaise

2 tbsp lemon juice

1 tsp agave syrup

1 unpeeled apple, cored and cut into cubes

1 cup celery, thinly sliced

1/2 cup raisins

1/2 cup toasted walnuts

2 large handfuls baby spinach

Whisk together the yogurt, mayonnaise, lemon juice, and agave syrup in a small bowl.

Place the apple, celery, raisins, walnuts, and spinach in a large bowl and toss with the dressing—simple and delicious!

SALAD NIÇOISE

This a French staple lunch in the summer. They even serve it in French schools at least once a week.

Serves 2
3 small red potatoes or a handful of tiny new potatoes, boiled until tender
2 hard-boiled eggs
Handful of green beans, trimmed
2 cups mixed lettuce leaves
2 medium tomatoes, quartered, or a handful of cherry tomatoes
8 black olives
1 can low-mercury tuna
6 anchovies (optional)
1 tbsp fresh flat-leaf parsley, chopped

Place the mixed salad leaves in a salad bowl and assemble all the remaining ingredients on top, finishing with the parsley. Dress with Gorgeously Green Dressing (page 63) or some really good olive oil and lemon juice.

CRUNCHY WATERCRESS DELIGHT

Peppery watercress and sweet orange make for a delightfully tangy combination. The crunch of the jicama and all the pretty colors make this one of my favorite lunchtime salads.

Serves 2
2 cups watercress, stalks removed
2 cups spinach
1 cup jicama, cut into matchsticks
1/2 cup sliced radishes
1/2 cup pitted and sliced black olives
1 orange, peeled, halved, and sliced

Assemble all the ingredients in a salad bowl and dress with a really good olive oil, lemon juice, and salt and pepper.

NUTTY COLESLAW

I make this sweet, satisfying coleslaw year-round. It's delicious with grilled meat or tempeh.

Serves 2
2 cups shredded red cabbage
1 cup shredded Napa cabbage
2 large carrots
6 scallions, chopped finely
3 tbsp toasted sesame oil
3 tbsp rice vinegar
1 tbsp agave syrup
1 clove garlic, minced
1 tbsp fresh ginger, minced
1/2 cup dry-roasted peanuts
1/2 cup raisins
2 tbsp sesame seeds

Combine the red cabbage, Napa cabbage, carrots, and scallions in a large bowl. Place the rest of the ingredients in a large jar with a screw top, shake vigorously, and dress the salad.

CORN AND BLACK BEAN SALAD

I'm a cilantro girl—I love it and grow it year-round. This is one of my favorite salads to use it in.

Serves 2
1 15-ounce can black beans
1 cup uncooked fresh or frozen corn
1 large tomato, diced
1 small red onion
2 tbsp finely chopped flat-leaf parsley
2 tbsp finely chopped cilantro
2 cloves garlic, minced
2 tbsp apple cider vinegar
1/4 cup olive oil
1/4 tsp ground cumin

¼ tsp ground turmeric
1 tsp agave syrup
Sea salt and freshly ground pepper to taste

Combine the beans, corn, tomato, onion, cilantro, and parsley in a large bowl.

Place the rest of the ingredients in a large jar with a screw cap, shake vigorously, and dress the salad.

ARUGULA AND RADICCHIO SALAD

This crunchy and refreshing salad works great on its own or with a piece of crusty olive bread or ciabatta.

Serves 2
2 tbsp extra-virgin olive oil
Juice of ½ lemon
1 tsp coarsely ground salt
¼ tsp ground pepper
2 cups chopped arugula
1 cup chopped radicchio
½ cup fresh Parmesan cheese cut into slivers with a vegetable peeler

Whisk together the olive oil, lemon juice, and salt and pepper in a wooden salad bowl. Add the arugula and radicchio and toss well. Top with the cheese.

LENTIL AND QUINOA SALAD

This packs a delicious protein punch—one of my favorites.

Serves 2 (make double; it keeps in an airtight container for up to a week)
½ cup quinoa
1 cup chicken or vegetable broth
1 cup green lentils
3 tbsp extra-virgin olive oil
Juice of 1 lemon
½ tsp salt
½ tsp black pepper
½ tsp ground turmeric

½ tsp paprika
½ cup chopped fresh basil
½ cup chopped flat-leaf parsley
½ cup pine nuts
½ cup raisins

Place the quinoa and broth in a small saucepan and bring to a boil. Cover, lower the heat, and simmer for 15 minutes, or until the liquid has been absorbed. Remove from the heat and set aside to cool.

Meanwhile, place the lentils in a medium saucepan and cover with 3 cups water. Bring to a boil, then lower the heat and simmer for 20 minutes, or until cooked through. Drain, rinse, and set aside to cool.

Make the dressing by whisking together the olive oil, lemon juice, salt, pepper, turmeric, paprika, basil, and parsley in a small bowl.

Combine the cooled quinoa and lentils in a large bowl, toss with the dressing, and mix in the pine nuts and raisins.

COCONUT CASHEW SALAD

You can serve this scrumptious salad either warm in the winter or cool in the summer. It makes a hearty lunch or a light dinner. It's delicious served with steamed brown rice.

Serves 2
2 tbsp virgin coconut oil
1 medium onion, chopped
1 thumb-size piece ginger, peeled and minced
1 red bell pepper, deseeded and chopped (if bell peppers aren't in season, substitute 1 large carrot, grated)
1 tsp curry powder
½ tsp turmeric
1 15-ounce can organic coconut milk
1 15-ounce can garbanzo beans, rinsed
1 cup raw cashews
1 Napa cabbage, chopped
2 tbsp chopped fresh cilantro

Heat the coconut oil in a medium sauté pan over medium heat. Add the onion and ginger and sauté until the onion is softened, about 5 minutes. Add the red pepper, curry powder, and turmeric and sauté for another 3 minutes. Add the coconut milk and garbanzo beans, bring to a simmer, and simmer for 5 minutes. Add the Napa cabbage and cashews and simmer for another 5 minutes. Spoon into bowls and sprinkle with the cilantro.

TOFU SALAD

This takes just a few minutes to prepare but the ingredients need time to marinate, so if you plan to eat it for lunch, make it right after breakfast.

Serves 4
MARINADE:
4 tbsp toasted sesame oil
5 tbsp cider vinegar
1 tbsp agave syrup
3 tbsp soy sauce
2 cloves garlic, minced
1 tsp fresh ginger, minced
1 pound extra-firm tofu (drain really well)
1 cup chopped white mushrooms
1 carrot, cut into matchsticks
1 red bell pepper, chopped
2 scallions, minced
2 cups finely shredded Napa cabbage

TOPPING:
1 cup chopped fresh cilantro
½ cup of peanuts, crushed
Lettuce leaves

Simply mix all the marinade ingredients together in a medium-size bowl. Add the tofu and vegetables and stir gently, making sure everything is coated. Cover with a large plate and let the whole thing marinate at room temperature for 2 or 3 hours.

Place lettuce leaves on individual plates and divide the salad among the lettuce cups. Garnish with the cilantro and peanuts.

GREEN LENTIL SALAD—3 WAYS

Since lentils are such an incredible source of protein and fiber and have so few calories, they make a great base for countless salads. Here are my favorite three.

GREEN LENTIL SALAD

The raisins in this salad give it a little sweetness and the pine nuts provide just the right amount of crunch.

Serves 4

2 cups green lentils
1/2 cup extra-virgin olive oil
1/2 cup lemon juice
1/2 yellow onion, finely minced
3 cloves garlic, minced
2 tsp ground cumin
1 tsp celery salt
1/2 tsp ground coriander
1/2 tsp ground turmeric
1 tbsp grated lemon zest
1/2 cup raisins
4 celery stalks, finely chopped
1/2 cup chopped fresh cilantro
2 tbsp crumbled goat cheese (optional)
1/2 cup toasted pine nuts

Wash, drain, and rinse the lentils, and put the lentils in a medium saucepan with water to cover. Bring to a boil, then reduce the heat and simmer for 25 minutes, or until tender. Drain and set aside to cool.

Whisk together the olive oil, lemon juice, onion, garlic, cumin, celery salt, coriander, turmeric, and lemon zest in a large bowl. Add the lentils, raisins, celery, and cilantro. Top with the goat cheese, if using, and the pine nuts just before serving.

GRILLED VEGGIE LENTIL SALAD

This is a summer variation of the Green Lentil Salad. The bright-colored peppers make it so pretty. It's great for entertaining.

Serves 2
1 cup green lentils, rinsed and drained
2 cups chicken or vegetable stock
1 cup chopped tomatoes
1 yellow or orange bell pepper, seeded and chopped
2 tbsp olive oil, plus more for drizzling
Salt and freshly ground black pepper
3 scallions, chopped
2 tbsp finely chopped fresh parsley
½ cup crumbled feta cheese
Balsamic vinegar

Preheat the oven to 400°F.

Combine the lentils and stock in a medium saucepan and bring to a boil. Reduce the heat and simmer for 20 minutes, or until tender. Drain and set aside.

Meanwhile, combine the tomatoes and bell pepper in a bowl and toss with the olive oil to coat. Season with salt and pepper and spread over a greased baking sheet. Place in the center of the oven and roast for 20 minutes, or until the vegetables are softened and lightly browned.

Transfer the roasted peppers and tomatoes into a large bowl and add the lentils. Mix in the scallions and parsley. Turn onto a serving dish and crumble the feta cheese over the top.

Drizzle a little olive oil over the dish and finish with a dash of balsamic vinegar.

POMEGRANATE, PEA, AND LENTIL SALAD

My friend Angela from England served this gorgeous salad for lunch. The pomegranate seeds embedded in it look like little jewels.

Serves 2
1 cup green lentils, rinsed and drained

2 cups water or vegetable stock
2 tbsp extra-virgin olive oil
1 red onion, chopped
½ cup frozen peas
⅓ cup chopped fresh parsley
⅓ cup chopped pomegranate seeds
Salt and freshly ground pepper

Combine the lentils and stock in a medium saucepan and bring to a boil. Lower the heat and simmer for 20 minutes, or until tender. Drain and set aside to cool.

Heat the olive oil in a medium sauté pan over medium heat. Add the onion, lower the heat, cover, and sauté until softened, about 5 minutes. Add the lentils, peas, parsley, pomegranate seeds, and salt and pepper to taste and give it a good stir. Cook gently for about 5 minutes, until the peas are cooked through. Do not put a lid on the pan or you will lose the lovely dual color of the pomegranate seeds and peas.

THAI CHICKEN SALAD

I love this salad—winter or summer, it's so tasty and a brilliant way to use up leftover chicken.

Serves 2
½ cucumber, deseeded, peeled, and cut into matchsticks
1 green chili, minced
1 tbsp minced fresh ginger
2 cloves garlic, minced
¼ cup lime juice
3 tbsp Thai fish sauce
4 tsp agave syrup
½ tsp sea salt
2 tbsp peanut oil
½ tsp chili oil
2 cups of chicken, deskinned and shredded
Cooked and cooled soba noodles

GARNISHES:
½ cup chopped fresh cilantro
½ cup chopped roasted peanuts

Combine all the ingredients except the chicken, noodles, and garnishes in a large bowl and leave to marinate for 30 minutes. Add the chicken, turn to coat well, and sprinkle the cilantro and peanuts on top. Serve with the soba noodles.

KATE'S RASPBERRY SALAD

My friend Kate is a wonderful cook and taught Lola and her best friend, Mira, how to cook an entire dinner party. This was one of the dishes:

Serves 2
1 cup fresh raspberries
1 cup walnut or extra-virgin olive oil
Rind of 1 orange, grated
1 cup fresh orange juice
3 tbsp raspberry vinegar
1 tsp honey
Sea salt and freshly ground black pepper
4 cups of lettuce leaves
1 red onion, thinly sliced
1 avocado, peeled, pitted, and sliced
4 ounces goat cheese, crumbled (optional)
1 cup coarsely chopped toasted walnuts

Press half the raspberries through a fine-mesh sieve into a screw-top jar, pressing on the solids to extract the juice. Add the oil, orange peel, orange juice, vinegar, honey, and salt and pepper to taste and shake well.

Combine the remaining raspberries with the lettuce, onion, and avocado in a large bowl. Toss with the dressing, and top with the goat cheese, if using, and the walnuts.

GRILLED EGGPLANT WITH YOGURT-MINT SAUCE

Since eggplants are pretty meaty, this dish is delicious for a light summer lunch, served with a toasted whole-wheat pita or some warm ciabatta bread.

Serves 4
1 cup plain yogurt
3 tbsp chopped fresh mint

2 tbsp fresh lemon juice
1 tsp curry powder
1 tsp peppered chili flakes
Salt and freshly ground black pepper
2 eggplants (1 pound each) cut into 1-inch rounds
¼ cup toasted sesame oil
2 tbsp crushed coriander seeds

Combine the yogurt, mint, lemon juice, curry powder, and chili flakes in a medium bowl. Season with salt and pepper to taste. The sauce can be made 1 day ahead; cover and refrigerate until ready to serve.

Prepare a grill over medium-high heat. Rub the eggplant slices on both sides with toasted sesame oil. Sprinkle with the coriander seeds and salt and pepper to taste. Grill until slightly charred, about 6 minutes per side. Serve with the yogurt–mint sauce.

MAYAN AVOCADO

When I was in Mexico, I ate a version of this recipe for lunch every single day. It's so light and delicious, perfect for a summer lunch.

Serves 1
1 cup finely chopped cantaloupe
1 tbsp chopped red onion
1 tbsp chopped fresh cilantro
Juice of ½ lime
1 large ripe avocado, cut in half and pit removed
1 whole-wheat or spelt tortilla, warmed

Combine the cantaloupe, onion, and cilantro in a small bowl and add the lime juice. Spoon into the hollowed-out avocado halves and serve with the tortilla.

SARDINE/TUNA LETTUCE CUPS

Sardines are so good for you. They contain omega-3 fatty acids, without the offending mercury. I was raised eating them but in the United States they are new to most people. It's a new taste, but give them a try and you'll be adding something incredibly beneficial to your diet. If you really don't like sardines, substitute with low-mercury tuna.

Serves 2
1 cucumber, peeled, seeded, and cubed
1 large tomato, seeded and cubed
1 small onion, minced
1 tbsp chopped fresh Italian parsley
1 tbsp chopped fresh mint
1 3.75-ounce can oil-packed sardines, drained and cubed
1 tbsp extra-virgin olive oil
1 tbsp lemon juice
1 tsp grated lemon zest
Salt and freshly ground black pepper to taste
4 to 6 outer romaine lettuce leaves

Mix all the ingredients, except the lettuce leaves, together in a large mixing bowl until thoroughly combined. Season with salt and pepper to taste, then spoon into the lettuce cups.

CURRIED CHICKEN CUPS

This is an easy and very satisfying meal that makes your chicken go further.

Serves 2
1 large chicken breast
2 cups chicken broth
1 cup plain yogurt
1 tsp ground ginger
2 tsp curry powder
4 celery ribs, diced
½ cup roughly chopped toasted almonds
Salt and freshly ground black pepper
1 cup seedless grapes
2 ripe avocados
3 tbsp flat-leaf parsley, chopped

Place the chicken breast in a small saucepan and cover with the broth. Bring to a boil, then reduce the heat and simmer for 15 minutes, or until cooked through. Remove from the pan, cool, and cut into cubes.

Combine the yogurt, ginger, and curry powder in a small bowl. Add the chicken, celery, grapes, and almonds and season with salt and pepper to taste. Spoon into the avocado halves and sprinkle with parsley.

TABBOULEH

This is a traditional Moroccan recipe that couldn't be easier. The most common mistake is to not use enough parsley, so be sure to use the full amount.

Serves 2
2 cups bulgur wheat or couscous (cooked)
2 large ripe tomatoes, chopped
4 scallions, trimmed and chopped
2 cups roughly chopped flat-leaf parsley
1/2 cup chopped fresh mint

DRESSING:
2 tbsp lemon juice
1 garlic clove, crushed
1/4 tsp ground cinnamon
1/4 tsp ground turmeric
Sea salt and freshly ground pepper
3 tbsp extra-virgin olive oil
Black olives

Prepare the bulgur wheat or couscous according to the directions on the box. Add the tomatoes, scallions, parsley, and mint.

To make the dressing, in a small bowl combine the lemon juice, garlic, cinnamon, turmeric, and salt and pepper to taste. Slowly whisk in the olive oil until emulsified. Toss the salad with the dressing and serve with the black olives.

PESTO

This is a basic basil pesto that can be used for many different recipes. You can drizzle it on soups, pizzas, or baked potatoes or serve it the classic way—in pasta. In the summer I make buckets of it with fresh basil from my garden. For variety try adding a few arugula leaves or 5 or 6 sun-dried tomatoes.

Serves 4–6 for pasta
2 cups fresh basil leaves
¾ cup pine nuts
1 cup grated Parmesan cheese
½ cup extra-virgin olive oil
Salt

Simply place all the ingredients in the blender and blend until it forms a thick paste. You should still be able to see tiny pieces of the pine nuts. If it's too thick, add a little more olive oil.

Add a little salt just before serving. You want to avoid adding salt before that, for it can darken the bright green color of the basil.

The pesto should keep for up to a week in an airtight container in your fridge.

SUMMER SOUPS

GORGEOUSLY GREEN GAZPACHO

This is a greens-rich version of this classic summer soup—my girlfriends love it!

Serves 4
2 cups chopped lettuce leaves
2 cups spinach leaves
2 cups chopped tomatoes
2 cups chicken broth
3 scallions, diced
1 medium cucumber, peeled and diced
1 tbsp chopped fresh parsley
½ cup sour cream, plus more to garnish (optional)
1 tsp chopped fresh mint leaves
½ tsp salt
½ tsp freshly ground black pepper

Put the lettuce leaves, spinach, tomatoes, and chicken broth in a blender and blend until smooth. Pour into a large bowl and add the rest of the ingredients. Chill for at least 1 hour before serving.

TRADITIONAL GAZPACHO

This is a traditional, robust gazpacho that should be made when all of the vegetables are ripe and in season—on a hot day, there is nothing more refreshing. My least favorite kitchen task would be skinning tomatoes, but it's totally worth the hassle for this amazing soup.

Serves 4–6
4 or 5 large ripe tomatoes, peeled, seeded, and chopped
1 red onion, thinly sliced
5 cloves garlic, minced
4 cups chicken stock
1 serrano chile, minced
2 cucumbers, peeled, seeded, and diced
1 red bell pepper, seeded and diced
1 ripe but slightly firm avocado, peeled, pitted, and diced
2 tbsp fresh lemon juice
2 tbsp medium-acid red wine vinegar
2 tbsp chopped fresh basil
2 tbsp chopped fresh Italian parsley
4 tbsp chopped fresh cilantro
Sea salt and black pepper in a mill
1/2 cup best-quality extra-virgin olive oil

Combine the tomatoes, onion, garlic, and stock in a large bowl and blend with an immersion blender until smooth. Stir in the rest of the ingredients except the olive oil. Chill the soup for at least 1 hour before serving. Remove from the refrigerator, stir, rest for 15 minutes, then drizzle the olive oil over the soup and serve.

ROASTED TOMATO SUMMER SOUP WITH BASIL PESTO

Roasting the tomatoes gives this soup a rich and unique flavor. The pesto is so pretty drizzled on top and perfect to be scooped up by a piece of crusty olive bread.

Serves 4
1 1/2 pounds medium tomatoes (make sure they are very red and ripe)
2 garlic cloves, minced

1 small bunch fresh basil leaves, chopped

3 tbsp extra-virgin olive oil

1 medium potato, peeled and roughly chopped

2 tsp tomato puree

1 tsp balsamic vinegar

Salt and pepper

4 tsp prepared or homemade pesto (page 282)

Preheat oven to 375°F.

Put the tomatoes in a large bowl and cover with boiling water. Leave for 1 minute, then carefully drain off the hot water. Skin the tomatoes using a clean cloth to protect your hands. Cut the tomatoes in half and place cut side up on a baking sheet. Place a little minced garlic, a basil leaf, and a few drops of olive oil on each tomato, place in the oven, and roast for 50 minutes, or until the edges are browned.

While the tomatoes are roasting, cook the potato in 2 cups water and the tomato purée for 15 minutes, or until easily pierced with the tip of a knife. Do not drain.

Scrape the tomatoes with all their juices into a food processor, add the potato-tomato water, and process until smooth. Season with salt and pepper to taste.

Gently warm the soup and divide among individual bowls. Top each bowl with 1 tsp pesto.

GARLICKY CUCUMBER SOUP

I just think this makes the perfect appetizer for a summer dinner party. It's refreshing, light, and so very easy to make.

2 cups Greek yogurt

1 cup cold chicken or vegetable stock

2 cloves garlic, crushed

2 tbsp chopped chives, and more for garnish

Juice of 1 lemon

1 large cucumber, peeled and grated

Salt and freshly ground black pepper

1 tbsp chopped fresh mint

Combine the yogurt, stock, garlic, chives, and lemon juice in a large bowl. Add the cucumber, stir well, and season with salt and pepper to taste. Chill for at least 1 hour.

Ladle into bowls and garnish with chives (and chopped chive flowers if you have them) and the chopped mint.

SUMMER FRUIT SOUP

I know this soup sounds rather weird, but do try it. Apart from being really easy to make, it is delicious and makes the perfect appetizer for a girls' lunch.

Take equal quantities of melon, cucumber, tomatoes, and avocado. Try to have all the pieces of fruit roughly the same size after they've been prepared.

Cut the melon in half and scoop out the flesh, or use a melon ball scooper. Peel the cucumber, cut lengthwise into 4 pieces, and then cut into cubes. Pop the tomatoes into boiling water for a minute or so and peel them. Peel and pit the avocado and cut into chunks.

Combine the fruits in a serving bowl or glass dish and sprinkle with a handful of fresh herbs, mint, parsley, tarragon, or whatever appeals to you.

Make a good, well-seasoned dressing of 1 part cider vinegar, 1 part olive oil, ½ tsp French mustard, ½ tsp sugar, and salt and pepper to taste.

Pour over the fruit and mix gently. Refrigerate for at least 3 hours. The amount of liquid will have increased a lot. Ladle the soup into pretty soup bowls.

Serve with a crunchy baguette to soak up the soup.

EVERY-SEASON SOUPS

GORGEOUSLY GREEN VEGETABLE SOUP

This easy soup is a staple in my kitchen. It is packed with veggie goodness and includes an easily digestible grain (barley) to fill you up. Served with whole-wheat bread, it's hearty enough for a family dinner. Think about making double quantities and freezing half of it for another time.

Serves 4
1 tbsp olive oil
1 medium onion, chopped
2 stalks celery, chopped
1 leek, chopped
1 tsp sea salt
1 tsp pepper

1 bay leaf

2 medium carrots, cubed

4 cups vegetable broth or 4 cups water with vegetable bouillon cube

¼ cup pearl barley

½ cup frozen edamame

1 cup broccoli, chopped into tiny florets

1 cup cauliflower, chopped into tiny florets

½ cup fresh or frozen and thawed corn

Chopped fresh parsley or mint to garnish

Heat the olive oil in a large stockpot over medium heat and add the onion, celery, leek, salt, pepper, and bay leaf. Sauté until the celery and leek are softened but not browned. Add the carrots and sauté for another 3 minutes. Add the vegetable broth and barley. Put a lid on the pot and simmer for 25 to 30 minutes. Add the edamame, broccoli, cauliflower, and corn and simmer for another 5 minutes or unti cauliflower is tender. Remove from the heat and serve garnished with handfuls of fresh chopped parsley or mint.

BLACK BEAN SOUP

2 tbsp olive oil

1 medium red onion, chopped

½ to 1 (depending on how hot you want it) jalapeño, deseeded and finely chopped

3 garlic cloves, minced

1 tsp ground cumin

½ tsp salt

2 15-ounce cans black beans, drained

1 quart vegetable broth

Greek yogurt to garnish

½ cup chopped fresh cilantro to garnish

Heat the olive oil in a stockpot over medium heat. Add the onion, jalapeño, garlic, cumin, and salt and sauté until the onions are tender, about 5 minutes. Add the beans and broth, cover, bring to a simmer, and simmer for 20 minutes. Serve with a dollop of creamy yogurt and a sprinkle of cilantro.

WINTER SOUPS

BRUSSELS SPROUT AND LENTIL SOUP

This was the winning recipe in the contest at www.gorgeouslygreen.com. It's the most delicious soup I have ever eaten, and every time I make it, all my neighbors beg for a bowl to take home. It's hearty enough for a winter lunch or a dinner party appetizer.

1 tbsp virgin coconut oil
1 medium onion, chopped
1 tbsp cumin, lightly toasted and ground
2 celery stalks, chopped
1 medium carrot, chopped
2 cups Brussels sprouts, topped and quartered
1 potato, peeled and chopped
2 cups (curly) kale, chopped
½ cup walnuts, chopped
½ cup green lentils
6 cups good-quality vegetable stock
Pinch of sea salt and freshly ground black pepper
1 tbsp Dijon mustard
½ cup Parmesan cheese, freshly grated
1 tbsp Worcestershire sauce
1 tsp walnut oil per bowl

Put the coconut oil in a large saucepan and add the onion, cumin, celery, carrot, and 2 tbsp water, and cover. Soften the ingredients over a low heat, then add Brussels sprouts, potato, kale, ¾ of the walnuts, lentils, and 4 tbsp water, and cover.

Once the kale has wilted, add the hot stock and season with the salt and pepper, and put the lid back on the pot. Gently simmer the ingredients until tender.

Add the mustard and liquefy the soup in a blender to the finest possible consistency.

Return the soup to the saucepan and add the Parmesan cheese. Adjust seasoning. You could add a tiny bit of Worcestershire sauce at this stage.

Serve with a swirl of walnut oil and the remaining walnuts, and some fresh spelt or rye bread.

FRENCH ONION SOUP

The caramelized onions give this classic soup a sweet, buttery flavor.

Serves 4
4 tbsp butter
3 tbsp olive oil
2 large onions, thinly sliced
2 cloves garlic, crushed
1 tbsp sugar
1 cup dry white wine
1 quart good stock (any type)
Salt and freshly ground black pepper
6 slices French bread cut diagonally 1-inch thick
1 clove garlic, peeled
6 ounces Gruyère or cheddar cheese, grated

Preheat the broiler.

Melt the butter with 2 tbsp of the olive oil in a heavy saucepan over medium heat. Add the onions, garlic, and sugar and keep stirring until the onions start to brown. Turn the heat down to very low and cook for about 15 minutes, until the onions are caramelized. Stir in the wine and stock, bring to a simmer, and cook at a low simmer for 30 to 45 minutes.

Meanwhile, brush the bread slices with the remaining tablespoon olive oil and toast under the broiler until brown. Rub one side with peeled garlic.

Ladle the soup into ovenproof bowls and float the pieces of toast on top. Sprinkle with the cheese and put under the broiler until cheese starts to melt.

CREAMY CARROT AND PARSNIP SOUP

This has got to be the most comforting soup on the planet. The parsnips give it a velvety texture. It's hearty enough for a winter lunch, or serve with a large salad and crusty bread for dinner.

Serves 4
1 tbsp olive oil
1 medium onion, chopped
3 celery stalks, finely chopped

1 tsp grated fresh ginger
½ tsp curry powder
Salt and freshly ground black pepper
4 medium carrots, peeled and chopped
2 medium parsnips, peeled and chopped
6 cups vegetable or chicken broth (or stock made from bouillon cubes)
4 tsp sour cream (optional)
Handful of chopped fresh parsley

Heat the olive oil in a large saucepan over medium heat. Add the onion and celery and sauté until softened, about 5 minutes. Add the ginger and curry powder and cook for 1 minute. Season with salt and pepper to taste and add the carrots and parsnips. Sauté for another 3 to 4 minutes, then add the stock. Cover the pan, bring to a simmer, and simmer for 30 minutes. Remove from the heat and cool for 10 minutes. Using an immersion blender, blend the soup until very smooth. Ladle into warmed soup bowls and top each with 1 tsp sour cream, if using. Garnish with the parsley.

RAINBOW CHARD AND COCONUT SOUP

This is super-easy, super-healthy, and super-inexpensive!

Serves 4–6
2 tbsp olive oil
2 medium yellow onions, chopped
1 clove garlic, finely chopped
2 cups chopped rainbow chard (stalks removed)
1 cup chopped kale (stalks removed)
1 quart vegetable stock
1 16-ounce can coconut milk
Salt and freshly ground black pepper

Heat the olive oil in a large saucepan over medium heat. Add the onions and garlic and sauté until softened, about 5 minutes. Add the chard, kale, stock, and coconut milk, bring to a simmer, and simmer for 10 minutes. Using an immersion blender, blend until smooth. Season with salt and pepper to taste and serve.

CREAMY PUMPKIN SOUP WITH BROWN RICE AND SWISS CHARD

With the rice, this is hearty enough for a cozy winter dinner.

Serves 4
2 tbsp butter
1 onion, chopped
2 cloves garlic, finely chopped
1 tsp ground cumin
1/2 tsp red chili flakes
7-ounce pumpkin, seeds and flesh removed, chopped into 1-inch cubes
3 cups chicken or vegetable stock
3 cups whole milk (vegan: soy milk)
Sea salt and freshly ground black pepper
1 cup chopped green Swiss chard, stalks removed
1 cup cooked brown rice
1/4 tsp ground cinnamon

Melt the butter in a heavy stockpot over medium heat. Add the onion and garlic and sauté until softened, about 5 minutes. Add the cumin and red chili flakes and cook for 2 minutes. Add the pumpkin, stock, milk, and salt and pepper to taste, and bring to a boil. Turn down the heat and simmer for 20 minutes, or until the pumpkin is tender. Purée the soup with an immersion blender until smooth. Add the chard leaves and simmer for 5 minutes. Spoon into warmed soup bowls, add a mound of rice to each bowl, and dust with a little cinnamon.

DIPS AND VEGGIE DISHES FOR SNACKS AND LIGHT LUNCHES

WHITE BEAN HUMMUS

This is an incredible dip for crackers, toasted pita bread, or crunchy veggies.

Serves 4 as a dip or small appetizer
1 1/2 cups white beans cooked, or 1 can drained and rinsed
2 large cloves garlic, finely chopped

2 tbsp fresh lemon juice
1 tbsp tahini
½ cup organic extra-virgin olive oil
Pinch of paprika
Salt and freshly ground pepper

Place the beans, garlic, lemon juice, and tahini in the bowl of a food processor, then blend until smooth. With the machine running, slowly add the olive oil through the hole in the lid until the mixture is emulsified. Season with the sea salt and pepper to taste, and sprinkle with the paprika.

TRADITIONAL HUMMUS

I have added a little fried onion to make this hummus extra-tasty; however, if you're pressed for time, you can leave it out and use canned garbanzo beans instead of the dried.

Since store-bought hummus is expensive, you can make your own for a fraction of the price, especially if you use dried beans.

Serves 4
1 cup garbanzo beans, soaked overnight with a pinch of baking soda
6 tbsp extra-virgin olive oil
½ large yellow onion, finely chopped
¼ tsp ground cinnamon
Juice of 1 1emon
2 large garlic cloves, crushed
4 tbsp tahini
Sea salt and freshly ground black pepper
1 tbsp pine nuts, lightly toasted
1 medium bunch of chopped flat-leaf parsley
½ tsp paprika

Rinse the soaked garbanzo beans under cold water, then place in a large saucepan and cover with cold water. Bring them to a boil, reduce the heat, and simmer for 1½ to 2 hours or until the skins are tender. Put to one side, keeping the beans in the water.

Heat 2 tbsp of the olive oil in a small skillet and sauté the onion on low heat until golden. Remove from the heat and add the cinnamon. Set aside.

Drain the garbanzo beans, keeping aside the cooking water, and blend in a food processor. If the mixture is too dry, add a little of the cooking water. When smooth, add the lemon juice, garlic, tahini, and the remaining olive oil. Add the salt and pepper and some more of the cooking water if needed.

Spoon the hummus into a bowl and sprinkle with the sautéed onions, pine nuts, parsley, and paprika.

Serve with raw veggies or warm pita bread.

TOMATO BRUSCHETTA

I am a massive fan of bruschetta in the summer. You can put so many different toppings on them and they are wonderful nibbles to offer your guests before dinner. Also enjoy them for a light summer lunch. The key is that you have to use good French bread or ciabatta. If there is a bakery in your grocery store, look for a freshly baked baguette or ciabatta loaf.

Serves 4–6
6 ripe in-season tomatoes
1 ciabatta or baguette, cut into 1-inch slices
1 clove garlic, peeled and cut in half
About 6 tbsp extra virgin olive oil
Handful of fresh basil leaves, torn
A few drops of good extra virgin olive oil
Salt and freshly ground black pepper
Rock salt

Place the tomatoes in a bowl, pour boiling water over them, and leave for 1 minute. Drain, then slip off their skins, holding the tomatoes with a kitchen towel. Finely chop the tomatoes and place them in a small bowl.

Heat a ridged grill pan until very hot. Place the bread slices on the grill pan on the diagonal and grill for about 1 minute on each side, until grill marks show. As soon as you take them off, rub one side of the toast with the cut side of the garlic and drizzle about ½ tbsp of olive oil on each slice. Arrange them on a platter.

Spoon about a tablespoon of tomatoes on each slice and top with some basil and a few drops of good olive oil. Crack some pepper and sprinkle a tiny pinch of rock salt onto each slice.

294 ~ THE *Gorgeously* GREEN DIET

BABA GHANOUSH

I sometimes make double quantities of this delicious dip and keep it for a few days in a sealed container in the fridge—that way, if I get hungry, I can just dip some crispy carrots or celery into it for an easy snack.

Serves 4–6
3 medium eggplants, cut in half lengthways
1 tsp plus 2 tbsp olive oil
2 cloves garlic, peeled
4 tbsp tahini
Juice of 2 lemons
½ tsp chili powder
1 tsp ground cumin
½ tsp ground turmeric
Salt and freshly ground black pepper

Preheat oven to 375°F.

Drizzle the eggplants with 1 tsp olive oil and bake on a baking sheet in the oven for an hour or until soft. Once they have cooled down, scoop out the flesh and put into a food processor along with all the remaining ingredients and blend until smooth. Add salt and pepper to taste.

SPICY CHICKPEAS

This is a delicious side dish that can be made any time of the year.

Serves 4–6
2 cups cooked garbanzo beans, either canned or soaked overnight
  and boiled
4 tbsp olive oil
2 tbsp white wine vinegar
Juice of 1 lemon
1 tsp ground cumin
1 tsp ground coriander
2 tsp paprika
1 tsp turmeric

2 tsp cinnamon
Salt and freshly ground black pepper to taste

Place the garbanzo beans in a large bowl. Add the oil, vinegar, and lemon juice and stir to coat. Add the remaining ingredients, toss to coat, and serve.

CRUNCHY NUT MIX

You can use a blend of whichever nuts you like most—I suggest raw almonds (no skins), pecans, walnut halves, peanuts, and macadamia nuts.

Since it takes awhile for the drying-out process, plan to make these nuts on a day when you're at home for the entire day—you don't want to leave your oven unattended. Make a double batch and store them in an airtight container.

4 cups mixed raw nuts
1 tbsp sea salt
1 tbsp tamari or soy sauce

Put the nuts in a bowl with the salt and cover with filtered water. Leave them at room temperature for about 8 hours or overnight and then drain and rinse.

Preheat oven to 250°F.

Spread the nuts over a baking sheet and bake in the oven for 2 hours.

Remove from the oven, cool, and store in an airtight container.

SPINACH TORTILLA

Packed with nutrients, this light tortilla is one of my go-to recipes when I'm in a hurry. You can make more of a meal of it with a green side salad and crusty olive bread.

Serves 2
2 tsp olive oil
1 large yellow onion, thinly sliced
1 cup fresh spinach leaves
3 medium eggs, beaten
1 ounce grated cheese (cheddar, goat, or feta)

Preheat the broiler.

Heat the olive oil in a small heatproof skillet over low heat. Add the onion and sauté for about 8 minutes, until lightly golden. Add the spinach and stir until wilted. Stir the eggs into the spinach and onion and cook for 8 minutes, or until almost set. Spread the grated cheese on top and put the pan under the broiler for 2 minutes, or until the top is bubbling and brown. Remove from heat and allow to cool before cutting into slices.

SUMMER DINNERS

EGGPLANT PARMIGIANA

I love this vegetarian "meaty" dish. I suggest baking the eggplant, instead of frying, because it's easier and the eggplant soaks up less oil. Double the recipe while you're at it and freeze one to save time.

Serves 4–6
3 medium eggplants, sliced lengthwise into ½-inch slices
2 tbsp olive oil
Salt and pepper
2 cups Easy All-Purpose Tomato Sauce (page 174) or 1 25-ounce jar
 organic tomato pasta sauce
Handful of chopped fresh basil leaves
2 cups shredded mozzarella cheese
½ cup grated Parmesan

Preheat the oven to 400°F.

Grease a baking sheet with olive oil. Place the eggplant slices on the baking sheet in one layer and brush with the olive oil. Bake for 20 minutes, or until lightly browned, turning once.

Grease an ovenproof dish and layer with the baked eggplant, tomato sauce, basil, and mozzarella cheese. Sprinkle the Parmesan cheese on top. Return to the oven and bake until bubbly and crisp on top.

QUINOA GADO-GADO

Gado-Gado is a traditional Indonesian dish with a peanut sauce dressing. I cook with quinoa whenever I can because it's easy to digest and full of protein. I also love its nutty taste.

Serves 4
4 cups cooked quinoa or brown basmati rice
3 cups baby spinach
1 cup finely shredded red cabbage

1 cup finely shredded Napa cabbage

2 carrots, cut into matchsticks

1 yellow or orange bell pepper, seeded and sliced

1 tbsp peanut oil

1 8-ounce package tempeh, sliced

1 tbsp virgin coconut oil

1 cup minced onion

1 tbsp minced fresh ginger

1½ cups smooth natural peanut butter

2 tbsp cider vinegar

2 tbsp tamari or soy sauce

1 tbsp raw honey

1 tbsp lemon juice

2 cups hot water

2 tbsp unsweetened shredded coconut

Arrange the quinoa on a beautiful platter and top with the spinach, followed by the red cabbage, Napa cabbage, carrots, bell pepper. In a small skillet, heat the peanut oil and fry the tempeh slices for 4 minutes on each side.

In a medium saucepan, heat the coconut oil over medium heat. Add the onion and ginger and sauté until softened, about 5 minutes. Add the remaining ingredients except the shredded coconut, and whisk until well blended. Bring to a simmer, then reduce the heat to low and simmer for 10 minutes, adding a little more water to thin it out if necessary.

Pour the sauce over the vegetables and tempeh and sprinkle with the shredded coconut.

FANCY CHEESY GRITS WITH BACON AND ARUGULA

I make this regularly for my southern husband who adores grits. The combo of Parmesan and bacon is irresistible, and the peppery arugula finishes the dish off to perfection.

Serves 2

4 strips nitrate-free bacon

2 cups water

½ cup yellow corn grits

¼ teaspoon salt

½ cup grated Parmesan cheese
2 cups arugula leaves
Extra-virgin olive oil for drizzling

Cook the bacon in a small skillet over medium heat until very crisp. Remove from the skillet to a paper towel to drain, set aside to cool, then crumble it.

Bring the water to a boil in a medium saucepan and slowly whisk in the grits. Add the salt. Reduce the heat and simmer for 5 minutes, stirring constantly so you have a creamy consistency. If the mixture is too thick, add a little more water and cook to desired consistency. Stir in the cheese and bacon. Remove from the heat and add the arugula to the pan. Cover with a lid and let stand for 3 minutes to wilt the arugula. Gently stir in the arugula and serve in warmed bowls with a drizzle of oil.

SHEPHERD'S PIE

This is a classic English dish and a wonderful and easy way to incorporate lamb into your diet. If you don't like the taste of lamb, you can always substitute ground beef.

Serves 4
1 tablespoon pure olive or canola oil
1 large yellow onion, chopped
2 medium carrots, cubed
1 clove garlic, minced
2 pounds ground lamb
2 tablespoons ketchup
2 tablespoons Worcestershire sauce
2 tablespoons vegetable stock
1 bay leaf
Salt and freshly ground black pepper, to taste
4 large russet potatoes, roughly chopped
1 tablespoon butter
½ cup whole milk
2 scallions, finely chopped

Preheat the oven to 325°F.

Heat the oil in a large, deep skillet over medium heat. Add the onion, carrots, and garlic and sauté until softened. Add the lamb, stirring to break up any lumps, and cook until lightly browned and no pink spots remain. Add the ketchup, Worcestershire sauce, stock, and bay leaf and season with salt and pepper. Bring to a simmer, then cover the pan, reduce the heat to low, and simmer for 15 minutes.

Meanwhile, place the potatoes in a large saucepan, cover with water, and bring to a boil. Boil until cooked through and a fork can pierce a potato without resistance, 15 to 20 minutes. Drain the potatoes and return to the pan. Mash the potatoes with a potato masher, then stir in the butter, milk, and scallions. Season with salt and pepper to taste.

Place the cooked lamb in a 3½-quart baking dish and cover with the mashed potatoes, spreading them evenly over the lamb. Place in the oven and bake for 30 minutes, or until the lamb is bubbling and the potatoes are lightly browned. Serve with cooked peas or steamed cabbage.

Lentil and Cauliflower Stew

On a winter evening, this cozy and nutritious dish always does the trick.

Serves 4
1 cup red lentils
1 cup finely chopped yellow onions
1 tbsp grated fresh ginger
2 garlic cloves, minced
½ tsp ground turmeric
3 medium potatoes, peeled and quartered
½ small head cauliflower, cut into florets
1 tsp salt
6 tbsp ghee (page 172)
1 tsp cumin seeds
½ tsp ground cayenne pepper
3 tsp lemon juice
2 tbsp chopped fresh cilantro
½ cup plain yogurt

Wash the lentils, drain, and put them in a stockpot or heavy saucepan with the onions, ginger, garlic, turmeric, and 3 cups of water. Bring to a boil, then reduce the heat and simmer for 15 minutes.

Add the potatoes, cauliflower, salt, and another 2 cups of water. Bring back to a simmer and cook for 15 minutes.

In a small skillet, heat the ghee over medium heat. Add the cumin and cook until lightly browned and aromatic. Add the cayenne, stir, and pour the ghee mixture into the stew. Add the lemon juice and cilantro. Top each serving with 1 tbsp yogurt and serve with brown basmati rice.

NATASHA'S WARM SCALLOP SALAD

My lovely friend Natasha always puts together the yummiest combinations of flavors. Here is her latest concoction, which has become a family favorite. It's perfect for an easy supper and uses farmed bay scallops, which are a good sustainable choice. This is one of the rare times that I use a microwave. I just can't turn on my oven for half an hour to cook one potato.

Serves 2
1 large sweet potato
Olive oil for brushing
Salt and freshly ground black pepper
3 cups arugula leaves
½ cup toasted pine nuts
12 small or 8 large bay scallops

DRESSING:
½ cup virgin olive oil
2 tbsp balsamic vinegar
1 tsp honey
Salt and freshly ground black pepper to taste

Preheat the broiler.

Pierce the sweet potato a few times with a fork. Place it in the microwave and microwave on high for 4 minutes, or until a knife slides in easily but the sweet potato is still firm. Remove from the microwave and set aside until cool enough to handle, then peel and slice ½-inch thick.

Place the sweet potato slices on a greased baking sheet and brush with olive oil. Generously sprinkle with salt and pepper and broil for about 3 minutes on each side, until browned. Leave the broiler on.

Meanwhile, whisk together all the dressing ingredients in a small bowl.

Toss the arugula, pine nuts, and dressing in a large bowl and mound it on individual plates. Top with the sweet potato slices.

Brush the scallops with a little olive oil, salt, and pepper and broil for about 2 minutes on each side, until just cooked through. Place the scallops alongside the salad and serve.

SHITAKE AND SEITAN STIR-FRY

Using a wok is a very energy-efficient method of cooking. This is very tasty, so make double if you are serving a hungry family.

Serves 2
3 tbsp hoisin sauce
1 tbsp plus 2 tbsp sesame oil
2 tbsp plus 2 tbsp soy sauce
1 tbsp rice vinegar
2 tbsp agave syrup
¾ cup vegetable broth
2 cloves garlic, minced
1 tsp minced fresh ginger
1 tbsp cornstarch
1 cup seitan, chopped into 1-inch pieces
3 to 4 scallions, chopped
1 red or yellow bell pepper
1 cup asparagus, chopped into 1-inch pieces
1 cup sliced shitake mushrooms
2 cups chopped broccoli

In a small saucepan over medium heat, whisk together the hoisin sauce, 1 tbsp of the sesame oil, 2 tbsp of the soy sauce, the rice vinegar, agave syrup, vegetable broth, garlic, ginger, and cornstarch. Bring to a simmer and simmer until the mixture thickens, 5 to 7 minutes, then remove from heat and set aside.

In a large wok or skillet, heat the remaining 2 tbsp sesame oil and 2 tbsp soy sauce over medium-high heat. Add the seitan and stir-fry until lightly browned, about 3 minutes. Add the scallions, bell pepper, asparagus, shiitakes, and broccoli and stir-fry another 2 to 3 minutes, until the vegetables are crisp-tender.

Add the sauce to the stir-fry, stir well, and cook for another 2 to 3 minutes, until the broccoli is softened. Serve over soba noodles if you like.

OVEN-ROASTED FLORENTINE PEPPERS

This is an all-time favorite of my family and friends. It can't go wrong and works very well as an appetizer for a dinner party.

Serves 4
4 red bell peppers
8 tbsp extra-virgin olive oil
4 medium tomatoes, cut in half
16 Kalamata olives
1 large bunch of fresh basil
8 anchovies (optional)
Sea salt and freshly ground pepper

Preheat the oven to 400°F.

Cut the red peppers in half, making sure you cut carefully through the stalk so it stays attached. Core and seed the peppers. Lay the pepper halves open-side-up on a large baking sheet.

Into each pepper half, place 1 tbsp olive oil, ½ tomato, 2 olives, 2 large basil leaves, and 1 anchovy, if using. Season with salt and pepper to taste. Place in the oven and bake for 45 minutes, or until the edges are shriveled and browned. Make sure you don't undercook—you want the peppers to slightly collapse.

Serve with bowls of arugula tossed in olive oil and lemon juice and topped with Parmesan shavings, and have a warm loaf of ciabatta or olive bread for dipping and mopping up the juices.

PORTOBELLO PESTO DELIGHT

This is my all-time favorite veggie recipe and I never make enough!

Serves 4
3 tbsp olive oil
2 cloves garlic, sliced
4 large portobello mushrooms, stems removed
4 tsp butter
3 tbsp vegetable or chicken broth
3 tbsp soy sauce

4 tbsp homemade pesto (page 282)
4 slices of goat cheese log

Preheat the oven to 375°F

Heat the olive oil in a large sauté pan with a lid over medium heat. Add the garlic and stir for a minute to soften. Place the mushrooms with their stalk side up in the pan and add 1 tsp of butter where the stalk was. Gently move the mushrooms around the pan for a couple of minutes to prevent sticking. Add the vegetable broth and soy sauce, put the lid on the pan, bring to a simmer, and simmer for 5 minutes.

Carefully take the mushrooms out of the sauté pan and place them in a baking dish. Put 1 tbsp of pesto and a slice of goat cheese into each mushroom. Cover with the liquid from the sauté pan. Put in the oven and bake for 10 minutes.

Serve with Creamy Mash (page 172).

TOLLEY'S SUMMER ZUCCHINI PIE

If you need to use up zucchini or find a creative way of cooking them, this recipe is seriously scrumptious, and children love it, too.

Serves 4–6
1 tbsp unsalted butter
1 cup whole-wheat bread crumbs
1 tbsp extra-virgin olive oil
1 medium onion, diced
2 garlic cloves, minced
2 medium tomatoes, seeded and diced
3 medium zucchini, quartered lengthwise and thinly
  sliced
1 tsp crushed fennel seed
1 tsp salt
Freshly ground pepper to taste
3 large eggs
1/3 cup milk
1 cup grated Swiss cheese
3 tbsp grated Parmesan cheese

Preheat the oven to 375°F.

Grease a pie plate with ½ tbsp of the butter, then sprinkle the breadcrumbs over the bottom and sides.

Heat the olive oil in a large skillet over medium heat. Add the onion and garlic and sauté for 10 minutes, or until browned. Stir in the diced tomatoes and sauté for 5 minutes. Raise the heat to high and add the zucchini, fennel, salt, and plenty of pepper. Cook until the zucchini is barely tender, about 5 minutes. Remove from the heat and cool at least 10 minutes.

Beat the eggs in a large bowl. Add the milk, then mix in the zucchini mixture. Pour half into the prepared pie plate, top with the Swiss cheese, then pour on the remainder of the mixture. Sprinkle the Parmesan cheese over the top.

Place in the oven and bake for 30 minutes, or until a knife inserted in the center comes out clean and the top is golden brown. Let sit 10 minutes before cutting. I find the pie looks much better about an hour after it comes out of the oven and has time to settle.

HERB-CRUSTED SALMON

I save this simple dish for when and if I can get locally caught wild salmon. I'll occasionally cook it with flash-frozen wild salmon, if I see a good bargain.

Serves 2
½ cup breadcrumbs
1 clove garlic, chopped
1 tbsp chopped fresh parsley
1 tbsp chopped fresh thyme
2 wild Alaskan salmon fillets
Salt and freshly ground black pepper
1 egg, beaten
2 tbsp olive oil
1 tsp butter

Combine the breadcrumbs, garlic, parsley, and thyme in a food processor and process until well mixed. Pour onto a large plate.

Season the fish with salt and pepper and dredge in the beaten egg and then in the breadcrumb mixture.

Heat the oil and butter in a large skillet over high heat until almost smoking, then carefully place the salmon fillets into the skillet. Cook for 4 minutes, until a nice brown crust is formed on the underside, then carefully turn the fillets over and cook until cooked through and nicely browned on the other side.

Immediately transfer the fish to warmed plates and serve with new potatoes, Hollandaise sauce, and cooked peas.

MEDITERRANEAN FISH OF THE DAY

This is an easy dish, which was given to me by the chef of a little seaside restaurant in Corsica. Use any white sustainable fish (such as black cod, tilapia, or whitefish).

Serves 4
3 tbsp good olive oil, plus more for drizzling
1 medium red onion
1 small red or yellow bell pepper, cored and sliced
2 tomatoes, chopped
1 tbsp capers
12 black olives
1 tbsp chopped fresh rosemary
2 cloves garlic, chopped
4 tbsp red wine
4 pieces of fish, each the size of a deck of cards

Preheat the oven to 400°F.

Heat the olive oil in a large cast-iron pan over medium-low heat. Add the onion and bell pepper and sauté for about 10 minutes, until softened but not browned. Add the tomatoes and the rest of the ingredients, except the fish. Pour into a gratin dish and lay the fish on the top. Season with salt and pepper and a drizzle of olive oil and bake for 10 minutes or until milky-white or opaque.

Remove from the oven and serve at room temperature with a good mixed green salad and some rustic bread cut into chunks to mop up the juices.

STUFFED BELL PEPPERS

Try to find small, evenly shaped bell peppers (any color) for this recipe. The smaller and younger they are, the more tender the flesh.

Serves 4
3 tbsp olive oil
1 medium onion, minced
2 anchovies, finely chopped
1 cup toasted whole-wheat breadcrumbs
1 cup ricotta cheese
½ cup grated Parmesan cheese
2 tbsp capers, drained and chopped
2 tbsp pine nuts
2 eggs, beaten
2 tbsp finely chopped fresh parsley
8 small or 4 medium-to-large bell peppers
½ cup water

Preheat the oven to 350°F.

Heat 2 tbsp of the olive oil in a medium skillet over medium heat. Add the onion and anchovies and sauté until softened, about 5 minutes. Transfer to a medium bowl and add the breadcrumbs, ricotta cheese, Parmesan cheese, capers, pine nuts, eggs, and parsley. Mix well to combine.

To stuff the peppers, slice off their tops (keeping the stalk on) and set the tops aside. Core and seed the peppers and cut a very thin slice off the base of each pepper so it can stand up straight. Stuff the peppers, set them in a deep baking dish, pour in the water, and drizzle the peppers with the remaining tablespoon olive oil. Bake uncovered for 45 minutes or until the tops are crispy and brown.

ARUGULA PESTO

I put pesto on a variety of vegetables, fish, and meat. There is nothing like homemade summer pesto, especially if you grow your own basil, which I recommend, for it requires no maintenance. Simply go to your local nursery in the late spring and buy about four or five plants (you'll use a lot), and plant in a sunny spot.

For pasta: Serves 2
1 cup arugula
1 cup fresh basil leaves, stalks removed
1 cup pine nuts
1 cup grated Parmesan cheese
1 cup good olive oil
Salt

Put all of the ingredients into the food processor and process, then scrape down the sides, process again, scrape one last time, and process again, making sure all the nuts and cheese are scraped from the sides of the bowl.

Transfer to a glass storage container with a lid. It will keep for up to 10 days in the refrigerator.

ANGEL HAIR PASTA WITH SCALLOPS

This dish is divine. The creamy scallops pair beautifully with the light, buttery angel hair pasta. Be aware that scallops require very little cook time, so watch carefully. When they turn from translucent to solid white, they're done.

Serves 4
6 tbsp extra-virgin olive oil
1 garlic clove, minced
1 small chili pepper, minced
16 small, fresh scallops, cleaned
5 ounces white wine
2 tbsp chopped fresh parsley
Salt and pepper to taste
13 ounces angel hair pasta, cooked al dente

Heat the olive oil in a large skillet over medium heat. Add the garlic, chili, and scallops and fry, stirring, for 2 minutes. Flip the scallops over and add the wine and stir until almost evaporated and the scallops are cooked through. Add the parsley and season with salt and pepper to taste. Toss the pasta into the scallop mixture and serve immediately.

THREE-MUSHROOM FETTUCCINE

This is my husband's signature dish and it is exquisite.

6 tbsp butter
1 small onion, chopped
2 ounces prosciutto, finely chopped
12 ounces mixed wild mushrooms (ideally a mixture of chanterelles,
** morels, and porcini mushrooms; if you can't find them fresh,**
** use dried and soak them in hot water for 15 minutes before**
** using)**
12 ounces egg fettuccine, cooked al dente
3 tbsp heavy cream
Salt and freshly ground black pepper
3 ounces Parmesan cheese

Heat the butter in a large skillet over medium heat. Add the onion and sauté until golden, about 5 minutes. Add the prosciutto and cook for 2 minutes. Add the mushrooms and sauté for 15 minutes, or until nicely browned. Add the pasta to the mushrooms along with the cream, salt and pepper to taste, and the cheese, and toss to evenly coat.

SALMON BURGERS

I use canned wild salmon because it's less expensive than fresh wild salmon and I can use it year-round. It's also an excellent way to get your omega-3s without having to worry too much about the mercury.

Makes 8–10 burgers
2 medium potatoes, peeled and cubed
2 6-ounce cans wild Alaskan salmon, drained
1 tsp lemon juice
1 small bunch chopped flat-leaf parsley
1 egg, beaten
Sea salt and freshly ground pepper
½ cup breadcrumbs
2 tbsp olive oil

Boil the potatoes in a pot of salted water for 15 minutes, or until tender. Drain.

Place the salmon in a bowl and mash up with the potatoes. Add the lemon juice, parsley, beaten egg, and salt and pepper to taste, and stir to thoroughly incorporate the ingredients.

Form the mixture into 8 to 10 patties. This is easier to do if you leave the mixture to firm up for an hour or so in the refrigerator.

Spread the breadcrumbs onto a plate and dip each patty lightly into them to give them a good coating.

Heat the olive oil in a sauté pan until it sizzles, turn down the heat a little, and add the patties, working in batches. Fry for 3 to 4 minutes on each side, until golden brown.

Note: You can make this recipe go further by adding another potato and upping the seasoning a little.

Serve with homemade tartar sauce (made with 1 cup mayonnaise, ¼ cup chopped capers, and 1 tsp chopped parsley).

TILAPIA VERACRUZ

This is my dinner of choice when I travel in Mexico. It's so healthy and delicious that I've started to cook it at home during the summer months when I can get organic, locally grown bell peppers. I love to cook this dish in an enamel casserole because the heat distributes evenly and cooks the vegetables beautifully. If you don't have one, use a heavy sauté pan.

Serves 2
2 large tilapia fillets
Salt and freshly ground black pepper
1 tbsp olive oil
1 medium onion, chopped
2 cloves garlic, minced
1 red bell pepper, seeded and chopped
1 yellow bell pepper, seeded and chopped
Handful of cherry tomatoes
1 tbsp chopped fresh cilantro
½ cup white wine
½ cup chopped flat-leaf parsley

Rinse the tilapia fillets, pat dry, season with salt and pepper, and set aside.

Heat the olive oil in an enamel casserole over medium heat. Add the onion and sauté until softened. Add the garlic and sauté for 1 minute. Add the bell peppers and sauté until softened, about 5 minutes. Add the fish, tomatoes, cilantro, and wine. Bring to a simmer, put a lid on the pan, and gently simmer for 10 minutes, or until the fish is cooked through.

Carefully place the fish onto serving plates and spoon the sauce over it. Garnish with the parsley and serve with brown rice or quinoa.

POACHED SALMON WITH DILL RAITA

I love to poach salmon—it's so clean and healthy and doesn't make my entire house smell fishy! This dish is simplicity and health on a platter. I really think it's best made with fresh fish, so keep your eye out during the summer for fresh wild salmon and treat yourself!

Serves 2
1/2 onion, peeled
2 wild Atlantic salmon fillets (each the size of a deck of cards)
1 tbsp chopped fresh dill
1/2 cup cucumber, very finely sliced (use a mandoline for paper-thin
  slices)
1 tsp lemon juice
1 tsp minced fresh mint
1 cup plain Greek yogurt
Sea salt and freshly ground black pepper

Bring a large pan of water to a boil over high heat. Add the onion and salmon fillets and half of the dill. Turn the heat down to very low so it is just simmering. The fish will cook very quickly, so time it carefully for 8 minutes, then remove from the water with a slotted spoon and place on warmed plates.

Combine the cucumber, lemon juice, mint, and remaining dill in a small bowl. Add the yogurt and season with salt and pepper to taste.

Place a large dollop of the raita alongside each salmon fillet and serve with tiny new potatoes and a mixed green salad.

LEMONY CHICKEN THIGHS

I love using chicken thighs, for they are much less expensive than chicken breasts and they are much tastier. Try to buy them at a butcher (not on a polystyrene tray) if possible.

Serves 2
4 bone-in chicken thighs with skin
2 lemons
1 tbsp olive oil
2 cloves garlic, minced
1 tsp celery salt
1 tsp salt
1 tsp black pepper
1 tsp dried thyme

Wash and pat dry the chicken and set aside in a small bowl. Whisk together the remaining ingredients and pour over chicken thighs. Place a plate on top of the bowl and refrigerate for at least an hour—the longer the better (fine to leave for a day!), turning them once to distribute the marinade.

When ready to cook, fire up a grill or preheat the oven to 400°F. Remove the chicken from the marinade and either grill, turning frequently, until cooked through, or place in an ovenproof dish and bake in the oven for 20 to 30 minutes. To check for doneness, sink a knife in close to the bone—if the juice runs clear, it's done; if the juice is still pink, put it back in oven for another 5 to 10 minutes and check again.

CITRUS ROAST CHICKEN

This is unbelievably easy, and remember, you can get at least one more meal out of your chicken (see Thai Chicken Salad, page 278).

Serves 4
1 large frying chicken
2 tbsp butter
1 tbsp olive oil
1 tbsp water
1 tbsp honey
Juice of 2 lemons
1 tbsp chopped fresh rosemary
Salt and freshly ground black pepper
2 large potatoes, peeled and cubed

Preheat the oven to 375°F.

Wash and pat dry the chicken and set aside. Combine the butter, olive oil, water, honey, and lemon juice in a small saucepan and heat over medium heat until the butter and honey are melted and the ingredients are well blended. Add the rosemary and season with salt and pepper to taste.

Place the potatoes in a large baking pan and cover with half of the lemon marinade, tossing to coat. Put the chicken in the middle of the pan and pour over the remaining marinade, massaging the marinade all over the chicken. Sprinkle 1 tsp salt and ½ tsp pepper over the chicken. Stuff the chicken with the squeezed lemon skins, put in the oven, and bake for 45 minutes to 1 hour, basting the chicken every 15 minutes, until the juices run clear when a knife is inserted close to the bone.

TRAY-BAKED LAMB CHOPS

This is so easy—everything just bakes in one pan, so it works well for a large family dinner.

Serves 2
1 cup olive oil
Juice of 2 lemons
2 cloves garlic, minced
1 tbsp chopped fresh rosemary
Salt and freshly ground black pepper
2 lamp chops (shoulder or leg chops work well)
4 medium carrots, sliced lengthwise
3 medium parsnips, sliced lengthwise

Whisk together the olive oil, lemon juice, garlic, rosemary, and salt and pepper to taste in a shallow bowl. Place the chops in the bowl and massage with the oil mixture. Cover the bowl with a plate and leave in the refrigerator overnight.

Preheat the oven to 400°F.

Put the chops with the marinade on a large baking sheet and add the carrots and parsnips, coating the vegetables with the marinade. Put in the oven and bake for 45 minutes.

VEGGIE BURGERS

It's hard to find a really great veggie burger recipe. My lovely friend Liz gave me this recipe and it's the best ever.

Serves 4
4 tbsp grapeseed or olive oil
1 medium onion, finely chopped
1 clove garlic, minced
2 large carrots, grated
2 medium zucchini, grated
1 16-ounce can garbanzo beans, drained
1 tbsp crunchy natural peanut butter
1½ cups whole-wheat breadcrumbs
1 tbsp chopped fresh parsley
1 tsp curry powder
1 tsp mixed herbs
1 egg, beaten

Heat 2 tbsp of the oil in a large skillet over medium heat. Add the onion, garlic, carrot, and zucchini and sauté until softened, about 5 minutes. Take off the heat and set aside to cool.

Place the garbanzo beans, peanut butter, breadcrumbs, parsley, curry powder, mixed herbs, and egg in a food processor and process for 20 seconds, or until the garbanzo beans are broken up and the ingredients are combined. Add the onion mixture and process for another 5 seconds (be careful not to overprocess).

Form the mixture into 8 patties, place on a plate, cover, and refrigerate for 30 minutes.

To cook the burgers, heat the remaining 2 tbsp oil in a skillet over medium heat. Add the patties in batches and cook for about 4 minutes on each side, until cooked through, well browned, and crisp.

TEMPEH HOT POT

I love this stew because you can leave it all day simmering in a slow cooker and come back to the delicious aroma in the evening.

1 tbsp peanut oil
1 medium onion, chopped
2 cloves garlic, minced
1 28-ounce can whole peeled tomatoes

1 15-ounce can garbanzo beans
1/2 cup white wine
2 tsp dried tarragon
1 tsp dried thyme
1/2 tsp paprika
1/2 tsp ground turmeric
2 bay leaves
3 cups vegetable broth
2 8-ounce packets of tempeh, cubed

Heat the peanut oil and fry the onions and garlic until soft. Place in the slow cooker with the rest of the ingredients and leave on a low setting for up to 10 hours.

VEGGIE FRITTATA

I like to make an extra-large frittata, since it's fantastic cold. You can take a couple of slices to work for lunch the next day—if it hasn't been polished off. It also makes a wonderful brunch dish for a large family or when you have guests.

Serves 8–10
3 tbsp olive oil
1 tbsp butter
4 small potatoes (preferably Yukon gold), diced
1 medium zucchini, diced
6 scallions, green and white parts, chopped
12 large eggs
1/2 cup whole milk
1/2 cup cottage cheese
Large handful of parsley or basil leaves (or a combination), chopped
Sea salt and freshly ground black pepper
1 cup crumbled goat cheese

Heat the oil and butter in a large skillet over medium heat until the butter is melted. Add the potatoes and cook for 7 to 10 minutes, until lightly browned. Push to one side of the pan, add the zucchini, and cook for about 5 minutes, until browned, and push to another side of the pan. Add the scallions and cook until softened, about 3 minutes. Mix all the vegetables together and distribute evenly over the pan.

In a bowl, whisk the eggs, milk, cottage cheese, and herbs together. Season with salt and pepper to taste and then slowly pour into the skillet. Reduce the heat to low and cook for 8 to 10 minutes, until the egg has set on the bottom.

Sprinkle the goat cheese over the top, transfer to the oven, and bake for 15 to 20 minutes, or until the top is lightly browned.

Cut into wedges and serve straight from the skillet with a green salad and some crusty whole-wheat bread.

WINTER DINNERS

TURKEY CHILI

This chili is packed with nutritious veggies for some extra antioxidant gorgeousness.

Serves 6–8
1 tbsp olive oil
1 yellow onion, chopped
2 cloves garlic, minced
1½ pounds organic ground dark turkey meat
1 tbsp chili powder
½ tsp ground turmeric
¼ tsp ground cinnamon
1 tsp salt
3 cups chicken or vegetable broth
2 tbsp tomato paste
2 tbsp Worcestershire sauce
1 15-ounce can kidney beans, drained
1 15-ounce can whole organic tomatoes
1 medium zucchini, cubed
2 medium carrots, grated
2 cups stemmed and chopped rainbow or Swiss chard
½ cup chopped fresh cilantro

Heat the olive oil in a large saucepan over medium heat. Add the onion and garlic and sauté for about 5 minutes, until softened. Add the turkey and cook for another 5 minutes, stirring to break up any lumps. Add the chili powder, turmeric, cinnamon, and salt and cook for 2 minutes. Add the broth, tomato paste, and Worcestershire sauce and stir to dissolve the tomato paste. Add the beans, tomatoes, zucchini, and carrots. Bring to a simmer, then reduce the heat to low and simmer for 15 minutes. Add the chard and simmer for another 5 minutes. Serve garnished with the cilantro.

VEGETARIAN CHILI

To make vegetarian chili, prepare as Turkey Chili above but omit the turkey, double the amount of kidney beans, and add one 15-ounce can of pinto beans.

MUSHROOM RISOTTO

I love to serve this risotto with a fresh bowl of arugula leaves dressed with olive oil and lemon juice.

Serves 4–6
1-ounce package mixed dried mushrooms
About 1 quart vegetable or chicken stock
1 tbsp olive oil
1 large onion, finely chopped
2 cloves garlic, finely chopped
4 celery stalks, finely chopped
1¾ cups risotto rice
2 wineglasses white wine
1 tbsp butter
Salt and freshly ground black pepper
Freshly grated Parmesan cheese

Put the mushrooms in a measuring cup and cover with 2 cups of hot water. Set aside.

Pour stock into a medium saucepan and heat gently. Keep warm over low heat.

In a large saucepan, heat the olive oil over medium heat. Add the onion, garlic, and celery and cook for about 5 minutes, until softened. Add the rice, turn up the heat, and stir until the rice looks translucent. Add the wine and stir until almost evaporated.

Now you are ready to add your first ladle of stock (you never leave a risotto—it needs to be nursed!). Keep stirring as you add more and more stock, waiting until each addition is absorbed until you add the next ladle. After 15 minutes, taste to see if the rice is cooked; if it needs a little more time, add a ladleful of the water that the mushrooms have been soaking in. The risotto is cooked when the rice is *slightly* al dente. Take it off the heat and stir in the mushrooms and butter. Season with salt and pepper to taste, spoon into bowls, and top with a generous dusting of cheese.

QUINOA WITH WHITE BEANS, SPINACH, AND MUSHROOMS

Serves 4
2 tbsp olive oil
1/2 yellow onion, chopped
2 cloves garlic, chopped
1 cup quinoa
3 cups vegetable stock
2 cups cooked great northern beans
1 cup sliced shiitake mushrooms
2 cups chopped spinach
Freshly grated Parmesan cheese

Heat the olive oil in a medium saucepan over medium heat. Add the onion and garlic and sauté until softened, about 5 minutes. Add the quinoa and cook for another minute. Add the stock, bring to a simmer, cover, and simmer for 15 minutes. Add the beans, mushrooms, and spinach and cook for another 3 to 4 minutes, stirring well. Spoon into bowls and top with cheese.

GARLICKY MUSHROOMS ON TOAST

One of my favorite comfort foods as a child was mushrooms on toast. I've added the eggs to make it a little more of a meal.

Serves 2
3 tbsp butter
2 thick slices sourdough bread
4 shallots, finely chopped
2 cloves garlic, finely chopped

10 ounces mixed mushrooms (such as cremini and shiitake),
   trimmed and sliced
Salt and freshly ground black pepper
2 tbsp sour cream or plain yogurt
2 tbsp finely chopped fresh parsley
2 fried or poached eggs

Melt 2 tbsp of the butter in a large skillet over medium heat and add the bread slices. Cook for about 2 minutes on each side, until lightly browned. Set aside and keep warm. Melt the remaining tablespoon butter in the skillet, add the shallots and garlic, and sauté for 2 minutes. Add the mushrooms and sauté for 8 minutes, or until softened. Season with salt and pepper to taste. Remove from the heat and add the sour cream and parsley. Serve the mushrooms on the toast and top with a fried or poached egg. Drizzle the pan juices over the top.

BEEF STEW

A beef stew is perfect in the winter. It's the least expensive way to eat beef since the cut is cheaper and you can make it go further. It's a good choice for a big family dinner.

Serves 6 to 8
2 pounds organic (preferably grass-fed) braising beef, cubed
1 tbsp all-purpose flour
Salt and freshly ground black pepper
2 tbsp olive oil
2 medium onions, chopped
2 large cloves garlic
2 carrots, diced
2 celery stalks, diced
3 medium mushrooms, sliced
1 cup red wine or beer
1 tbsp Wizard's Vegan Worcestershire Sauce (see Resources, page 341)
3 cups beef broth
1 tsp dried mixed herbs
1 bay leaf
1 tbsp apricot jam

Preheat the oven to 325°F.

Put the beef in a resealable plastic bag with the flour and salt and pepper to taste and shake until evenly coated.

Heat the olive oil in a large skillet over medium-high heat. Sauté the onions and garlic until soft. Remove from pan and set aside. Add meat to the pan and brown all over. Transfer to a large Dutch oven and sprinkle with the rest of the flour from the bag. Stir well and add sautéed onions and the remaining ingredients. Bring to a simmer, then cover with a tight-fitting lid. Transfer to the oven and cook for 2 hours. Remove the cover, stir, and taste a little of the gravy to check if it needs more seasoning. Return to the oven and cook for another hour. The meat should be soft and tender. Spoon onto warmed plates and serve with Creamy Mash (page 172).

Quinoa Pasta with Goat Cheese and Walnuts

I'm a big fan of quinoa pasta, as it is much higher in protein than wheat pasta and it has a delicious nutty flavor. Be really careful not to overcook it, as it can turn mushy if cooked too long. If you cannot find quinoa pasta, use whole-wheat pasta instead.

Serves 4
1 cup walnut halves
4-ounce goat cheese, crumbled
1 8-ounce box quinoa pasta (spaghetti, fettuccine, or penne)
1 tbsp chopped flat-leaf parsley
2 tbsp freshly grated Parmesan cheese

Preheat the oven to 375°F.

Place the walnuts on a baking sheet, place in the oven, and toast for about 10 minutes, turning once, until lightly browned. Remove from the oven, cool, and chop. Place in a large serving bowl along with the crumbled goat cheese.

Cook the pasta according to directions on the package and roughly drain, keeping a bit of water in the bottom of the pan. Add the drained pasta and cooking water to the serving bowl and toss with the walnuts and cheese. If the cheese seems a little thick, stir in ¼ cup of the cooking water. Add the parsley and serve topped with the Parmesan cheese.

VIETNAMESE CHICKEN NOODLE HOT POT

My mother makes this rejuvenating hot pot in the winter and there's never a single drop left. It is a wonderful and easy dish to serve to guests or just for the family.

Serves 4
4 ounces thin rice noodles
5 cups chicken stock
1/2 cup coconut milk
2 tbsp lime juice
2 chicken breasts, thinly sliced
1 tbsp peanut oil
3 large cloves garlic, finely chopped
2 poblano chilies, seeded and minced
Thumb-size piece of fresh ginger, minced
Handful of bean sprouts
Handful of fresh cilantro leaves

Cook the noodles according to directions on the package, rinse, and cool.

Heat the stock, coconut milk, and lime juice in a stockpot. When just coming to a boil, take off the heat and add the chicken.

Heat the oil in small skillet over medium heat. Add the garlic, chilies, and ginger and sauté for 2 minutes, or until softened, and add to the broth. Return the chicken and broth to the heat, bring to a simmer, and simmer for 5 minutes Add the bean sprouts and cilantro, ladle into individual bowls, and serve.

MILD VEGETABLE CURRY

I absolutely love a warming curry in the winter. This is a great recipe; you can use up a lot of your leftover veggies—those annoying two carrots that are rolling around in the bottom drawer of your fridge can be put to good use.

Serves 4
2 tbsp coconut oil
1 onion, chopped
1 tsp curry powder
2 4-ounce cans coconut milk

1 head cauliflower, chopped
2 carrots, chopped
1 parsnip, chopped
Handful of spinach, chopped
1 cup sliced mushrooms
1 bunch cilantro, stems removed and chopped

Heat the coconut oil in a large saucepan over medium heat. Add the onion and sauté until softened, about 5 minutes. Add the curry powder and cook for 1 minute. Add the coconut milk and vegetables. Simmer on a low heat for 20 minutes, stirring every now and then. Test the vegetables to see if soft, then remove from heat and serve with basmati rice and top with the cilantro.

LENTIL DHAL

This is a traditional Indian side dish that is comforting and highly nutritious. It's delicious eaten on its own or with rice.

Serves 4 as a side dish
1 cup yellow split peas, uncooked
2 cups water or vegetable broth
1 tsp ground turmeric
¼ tsp cayenne pepper
½ tsp salt
1 tbsp ghee or olive oil
1 onion, finely chopped
1½ tsp cumin, whole seeds or ground
2 whole cloves
Salt and pepper to taste

In a large pot, combine the split peas and water or vegetable broth over medium heat. Bring to a low simmer and add the turmeric, cayenne, and salt. Cover and cook for 30 minutes, stirring occasionally.

In a medium skillet, melt the ghee over medium heat. Add the onion, cumin, and cloves and cook for 4 to 6 minutes, until the onion is softened. Add the onion and spices to the split peas and simmer for 5 minutes. Season with salt and pepper to taste.

STUFFED POTATOES

This is a great, filling supper that is really easy to prepare for a hungry family. When I am baking potatoes, I like to make use of the energy that I am using by baking at least one other thing at the same time. Homemade granola is a perfect choice, as I can always use some more and the oven temperature is the same as for this recipe.

Serves 2
2 large potatoes
Salt
3 slices nitrate-free bacon (optional)
1 cup small broccoli florets
1 tbsp butter (optional)
½ cup grated cheddar cheese

Preheat the oven to 375°F.

Wash the potatoes and sprinkle them all over with salt. Prick them with a fork in a few places, place on a baking sheet, and bake for 50 minutes, or until easily pierced with a knife.

Meanwhile, you can prepare your granola, cake, cookies, or whatever else you are going to cook, or simply move ahead with the rest of this recipe.

Cook the bacon in a cast-iron skillet over medium-high heat until crisp.

Steam the broccoli until just tender—be careful not to overcook, as you want it to have a bit of a bite.

When the potatoes are ready, cut them in half and scoop the flesh into a bowl. Mash it up with the butter if you are that way inclined. Crumble up the bacon and mix gently with the potato mixture along with the broccoli. Spoon the mixture back into the potato skins and sprinkle the grated cheddar over the top. Put them back in the oven for another 10 minutes, or until heated through and the cheese is bubbly.

MEATBALLS WITH TOMATO SAUCE

This is a really delicious and economical recipe. I often make double quantities and freeze half.

Serves 4–6
3 slices whole-wheat bread, crusts removed and processed into crumbs
1 pound ground beef or lamb

1 large egg
2 tbsp all-purpose flour, plus more for dusting
2 cloves garlic, minced
1 large onion, minced
Handful of chopped parsley
1 tsp dried mixed herbs
1 tsp ground cumin
Salt and freshly ground black pepper
Olive oil

Soak the breadcrumbs in a bowl with a little water, then squeeze dry.

Combine all the ingredients very well in a large bowl.

With wet hands, form the mixture into balls (using about 1 tbsp for each). You should have about 16.

Spread some flour over a shallow plate and roll the meatballs around so you'll have a good crust when cooked.

Heat olive oil in a large skillet over medium heat. Add the meatballs and cook for about 6 minutes, stirring, until browned and cooked through. Transfer to a warm dish.

Serve with Easy All-Purpose Tomato Sauce (page 174) and lots of noodles or other pasta.

COZY COTTAGE PIE (VEGETARIAN)

Bursting with goodness, this is one of my favorite comfort foods. It makes a great nutritious family meal and I have to confess that my daughter loves to eat it with tomato ketchup—why not?

Serves 6
2 large sweet potatoes or yams, cut into 1-inch chunks
2 tsp butter, plus more for greasing
Salt and freshly ground black pepper
2 cups broccoli florets plus 1 cup peeled and chopped stems
1 cup chopped parsnips
1 cup sliced brown mushrooms
2 tsp Worcestershire sauce
1 large egg white

2 cups ricotta cheese

½ cup crumbled feta cheese

¼ cup buttermilk (you can throw the rest of the carton into a smoothie)

1 tsp Dijon mustard

½ tsp mixed dried Italian herbs

2 tbsp whole-wheat breadcrumbs (make in the food processer out of the leftover end of a loaf)

2 tsp grated Parmesan cheese

Preheat the oven to 400°F.

Cook the sweet potatoes in boiling salted water to cover for 15 minutes or until soft when pierced with a knife. Drain and mash. Add the butter, 1 tsp salt, and ½ tsp pepper. Set aside.

Steam the broccoli and parsnips for 6 to 8 minutes, until tender, adding the mushrooms for the last minute. Place the vegetables in a bowl, add the Worcestershire sauce, and season with salt and pepper to taste.

Combine the ricotta cheese, egg white, feta cheese, and buttermilk in a food processor and process until smooth. Add the mustard, Italian herbs, and a pinch of salt.

Grease a heatproof casserole with a little butter and spread the vegetable mixture over the bottom. Spoon the ricotta mixture on top, followed by the yams. Sprinkle with the breadcrumbs and Parmesan cheese.

Place the casserole in the oven and bake uncovered for about 30 minutes, until bubbling and the top is browned.

DESSERTS

PEACHES ROSEBUD

I made this for my friend Rosebud's birthday dinner—it's an old recipe and one of the best ways of eating peaches because it brings out their flavor so beautifully. If you like, you can top each peach with a teaspoon of mascarpone cheese or whipped cream.

Serves 6

6 large peaches

2 tbsp agave syrup

3 cups water

1 tsp vanilla extract

2 cups raspberries
1 tbsp sugar
A few mint leaves dragged through a bit of sugar

Put the peaches in a pitcher or bowl and pour a kettle of boiling water over them. Count to 10 slowly (10 seconds), then drain the peaches, peel them, and slice in half.

Combine the agave syrup, water, and vanilla in a large saucepan over medium heat. Bring to a simmer and add the peaches. Cover, reduce the heat, and poach the peaches for 8 minutes or until soft all the way through.

Remove the peaches from the liquid and carefully arrange them into a shallow serving dish.

Put the raspberries and sugar in a blender and blend until smooth.

Pour the glorious red mixture over the peaches and decorate with the mint leaves.

Pomegranate, Banana, and Ginger Brûlée

This stunningly delicious dessert takes crème brûlée to the next level.

Serves 4
4 egg yolks
3 ounces granulated sugar
2 cups heavy cream
1 cup milk
2 tsp ground ginger
1 banana, sliced
2 pomegranates, seeds scooped out
1 tbsp dark brown sugar

Preheat the oven to 300°F.

Whisk the egg yolks and granulated sugar together in a large bowl. Very gently heat the cream and milk with the ginger in a medium saucepan until almost boiling (about 180°F). Combine the banana and pomegranate seeds and spoon into the bottom of 4 small ramekins. Slowly whisk the cream mixture into the egg mixture, then pour the mixture back into the rinsed-out saucepan. Stir over low heat for about 5 minutes, until thickened. Pour into the ramekins to cover the fruit.

Make a water bath by placing ramekins in a large baking dish. Fill the dish with warm water until the water is halfway up the sides of the ramekins. Place in the oven and bake for 50 minutes, or until almost set when gently shaken. Cool completely, then refrigerate for at least 3 hours or overnight.

Just before serving, preheat the broiler. Sprinkle the dark brown sugar over the top of the brûlées and broil until the sugar melts and browns.

STEAMED CHOCOLATE SPONGE

My mother used to make this good old-fashioned recipe for a Sunday lunch treat. It will always wow your dinner guests.

Serves 4
1 stick butter
1/2 cup sugar
2 eggs, beaten
1 cup self-rising flour
2 tbsp cocoa powder mixed with 2 tbsp milk

CHOCOLATE SAUCE:
2 tbsp unsalted butter
4 ounces dark chocolate, broken into squares
2 tbsp heavy cream

Grease a 3–4-cup pudding bowl.

In a large bowl, beat the butter and sugar until light and fluffy. Add the eggs one at a time, beating well between each addition. Sift the flour over the mixture and fold in lightly. Add the cocoa and milk mixture and spoon into the pudding bowl.

Cover with wax paper and a sheet of foil large enough to allow for expansion and tie with kitchen string.

Put the pudding bowl in a large saucepan two-thirds filled with hot water. Cover and steam for about 1 1/2 hours, topping up with more hot water if necessary.

While the pudding is steaming, make the sauce: Put the butter and chocolate in a heatproof bowl set over a pan of simmering water and stir until the chocolate is melted. Beat in the cream.

To serve, remove the wrapping from the pudding and turn out onto a warmed serving dish.

Pour the hot chocolate sauce over the pudding and serve.

FLOURLESS CHOCOLATE CAKE (SCANDINAVIAN)

I love chocolate and so I had to include this recipe from my homeland—this is simply to die for!

Serves 12
12 ounces semisweet chocolate
⅓ cup milk
⅓ cup butter
4 eggs, separated
1 scant cup sugar
⅓ cup ground almonds
1 tsp baking powder

Preheat the oven to 350°F.

Grease a 9-inch cake pan, line with parchment paper, and grease the parchment.

Break the chocolate into small pieces. Place in a heatproof bowl and add the milk and butter. Place over a pot of simmering water and stir until the chocolate is melted.

In a large bowl, beat the egg yolks with half of the sugar and add to the melted chocolate mixture. Fold in the ground almonds and baking powder.

In a separate bowl, beat the egg whites with an electric mixer until frothy. Gradually add the remaining sugar, beating until stiff peaks form. Carefully fold the beaten egg whites into the chocolate mixture.

Spoon the batter into the cake pan and bake for 40 minutes, or until a wooden pick inserted into the center comes out clean. Carefully turn pan upside down to release cake on to a wire rack to cool. Serve with whipped cream.

LITTLE CHOCOLATE POTS

I love to make this for special dinner parties. You can serve it in pretty sherbet glasses, coffee cups, or any kind of little pot.

Makes 6 little pots
6 ounces dark chocolate
½ cup strong black coffee
1 tbsp unsalted butter, at room temperature

3 eggs, separated*
2 tbsp dark rum or 3 to 4 drops vanilla extract

Break the chocolate into pieces and put it into a saucepan with the coffee. Place over low heat and melt slowly to a thick cream, stirring occasionally. Remove from the heat and beat in the butter, then beat in the egg yolks one at a time. Add the rum.

In a large bowl, whisk the egg whites to stiff peaks and stir into the chocolate mixture using a metal spoon. Pour into small pots or pretty glasses, cover, and chill overnight before serving.

PAVLOVA

This recipe originated in Australia—a chef in Adelaide made it for the famous ballerina Anna Pavlova. My mother, who is famed for her version, taught me to make it when I was little.

Serves 6
2 tsp cornstarch
2 tsp white wine vinegar
1 tsp vanilla extract
4 egg whites
8 ounces superfine sugar

TOPPING:
10 ounces heavy cream
3½ cups raspberries
1 tbsp confectioners' sugar, plus more for dusting

Preheat the oven to 300°F.

Line a baking sheet with a sheet of parchment paper or a silicone mat. Lightly grease it and draw a circle on it with an upturned can approximately 8 inches in diameter.

Mix together the cornstarch, vinegar, and vanilla in a small bowl.

In a large bowl, beat the egg whites until they form soft peaks, then gradually add the superfine sugar, whisking all the time, until fairly stiff. Using a metal spoon,

---

*You should be fine using raw eggs as long as they are organic. The risk of *Salmonella* is practically nil in those kinds of eggs.

fold in the cornstarch mixture, then spoon the meringue mixture onto the baking sheet. Swirl it around, making a small dent in the middle.

Place in the oven and bake for 1 hour, then turn the oven off and leave to cool in the oven. The meringue base will keep for a week in an airtight container.

When you are ready to serve, transfer to a serving plate, whip the cream until it just holds its shape, and spoon the cream on the top of the meringue base. Cover with 3 cups of the raspberries and dust with confectioners' sugar. For the finishing touch, take the remaining ½ cup raspberries, blend with 1 tbsp confectioners' sugar, and drizzle over the top.

LINDA'S APPLE CRUNCH

This is a great recipe for using up stale bread, and kids love it!

Serves 6
4 large cooking apples, peeled, cored, and sliced
¼ cup light brown sugar
2 tbsp water
1 stick butter
6 slices white bread or brioche, cut into quarters
2 tbsp dark brown sugar
Yogurt or crème fraîche to serve

Preheat the oven to 375°F

Put the apples, light brown sugar, and water in a medium saucepan over medium heat. Cook gently, stirring occasionally for about 5 minutes or until softened. Transfer to a shallow ovenproof dish. Melt the butter in a small saucepan and pour onto a plate. Briefly dip both sides of each slice of bread into the butter and place them in overlapping layers over the apple. Sprinkle with the dark brown sugar and bake for 30 minutes, or until browned and crisp on top.

Serve with yogurt or crème fraîche.

BAKED APPLES

I was raised on baked apples, so for me they are an absolute comfort food. I love that something so healthy can be so satisfying.

330 ~ THE Gorgeously GREEN DIET

Serves 4
4 large Granny Smith apples
1 tsp butter, softened
1/2 cup raisins
1/2 cup chopped walnuts
1/2 cup apple juice
1/4 cup raw honey
Plain yogurt and cinnamon to serve

Preheat the oven to 375°F.

Peel and core the apples. Using your hands, grease the apples with the butter.

Stuff the center of each apple with the raisins and walnuts. Put the apples in a shallow ovenproof dish, pour the apple juice around them, and drizzle the honey over the top.

Place in the oven and bake for 30 to 40 minutes, until soft when pierced with a fork. Remove from the oven and serve with a spoonful of yogurt and a sprinkle of cinnamon.

DRINKS

ICED CAFÉ LATTE

1 cup cold almond milk
1/4 cup freshly brewed coffee (keep some coffee from breakfast in
  the fridge), decaf or regular optional
1/2 cup crushed ice
1/2 tsp vanilla extract
Stevia to taste

Put all the ingredients in a blender and process until almost smooth.

GORGEOUSLY GREEN SODA

Instead of soda, I make my own sparkling water with my Soda Club Fountain (www .sodaclubusa.com), which is a wonderful green accessory for your kitchen. Then I add organic fruit juices and, if I want to be fancy, I add a sprig of lavender and some torn-up mint leaves. This will end up saving you a great deal of money and help you and your family to do away with hideously unhealthy sodas.

SECTION NINE

Resources

ONLINE RESOURCE GUIDE

For an up-to-the-minute guide, where you can find all the following resources in one place, visit www.gorgeouslygreen.com/catalog.

DAIRY PRODUCTS

Milk, butter, cream, cottage cheese: It's not an easy task to find the raw and un-homogenized milks that I recommend. You may have to look further than your local grocery store. However, I really suggest that you make the effort if you and your family are daily milk drinkers.

RAW MILK
If you want to find the best supplier of raw milk in your area, go to www.realmilk.com and type in your zip code.

ORGANIC NONHOMOGENIZED MILK
My favorite dairy is called Straus Family Farm (www.strausfamilycreamery.com). The quality of the milks, creams, butters, and yogurts is exceptional. None of their milk is homogenized and they use only glass bottles.

Organic Valley is also a great organic milk supplier (www.organicvalley.coop). They carry nonhomogenized whole milk, but they don't use glass bottles. They have a huge selection of dairy products, including excellent organic butter. Many large grocery stores carry this brand, and on their Web site they always have coupons!

The following big-chain grocery stores either have their own generic, organic brand or carry a large selection of organic items:

Albertsons (Wild Harvest)
Big Y
Kroger/Ralphs (Private Selection)
Meijer (Meijer Organics)
Publix
Safeway/Vons ("O" Organics)
Shaw's (Wild Harvest)
ShopRite (ShopRite Organics)
Stop & Shop (Nature's Promise)
Super Fresh
Wegmans (Wegmans Organic)
Giant (Nature's Promise)
Costco (Kirkland Signature)
Fred Meyer
Target (Archer Farms)
Whole Foods (365)

KEFIR

This is a must-have product for the Gorgeously Green Girl. It is satisfying and delicious and works really well for this diet.

My favorite kefir is Nancy's Organic Kefir (www.nancysyogurt.com). It is sweetened with organic agave syrup and is packed with real organic fruit. The blackberry kefir is out of this world.

Lifeway Foods (www.lifeway.net), available in large grocery chains, also carries a good line of kefir products, and you can download and print coupons that will be accepted in most grocery stores.

YOGURT

Stonyfield Farm is the leader in the organic yogurt business. Their yogurt is widely available in large grocery chains and they have many green initiatives. Look for their plain whole-milk yogurts (www.stonyfield.com).

If you like Greek yogurt, Oikos yogurt (www.oikosyogurt.com) is heavenly. Oikos's parent company is Stonyfield.

Other brands I like:

Brown Cow (www.browncowfarm.com) (offers coupons)
Rachel's (www.rachelsdairy.com)
Redwood Hill Goat Yogurt (www.redwoodhill.com)
Fage (www.fageusa.com)

I also recommend all of the large chain-store-brand organic plain yogurts.

CHEESE AND DAIRY ALTERNATIVES

I recommend only dairy alternatives that contain no added sweeteners, thickeners, emulsifiers, or any other kind of unhealthy additive. I suggest the following, all of which are available at most health food stores.

Follow Your Heart Vegan Gourmet (www.followyourheart.com)
Lisanatti almond and rice cheese (www.lisanatticheese.com)
Soya Kaas cheese

BUTTER

To find raw butter, you can go to www.westonprice.org and find out where your local supplier is.

Look for large chains' organic brands of butter. I also recommend:

Straus Family Creamery Butter
365's organic butter (Whole Foods)
Organic Valley Cultured Butter
Trader Joe's organic sweet cream butter
Kerrygold butter (www.Kerrygold.com)

MEAT

If you buy meat, the very best thing you can do is to find a local farm and strike up a relationship or join a community supported agriculture scheme—this way your meat won't have to travel too far and won't have to be heavily packaged, and you will have the satisfaction of being able to put a face to the person who reared the meat that you are eating.

If you want to buy from your grocery store, here are the brands that I recommend:

Niman Ranch (www.nimanranch.com) carries organic beef, chicken, and pork, and uses traditional and humane methods to raise their animals.

Coleman Natural beef and lamb (www.colemannatural.com)

Shelton's Poultry (www.sheltons.com)

Rocky Range chicken (www.petalumapoultry.com)

Rosie Organic Free Range chicken (www.petalumapoultry.com)

Applegate Farms (www.applegatefarms.com) is a great brand for deli meats, including sliced turkey, chicken, ham, and salami.

Albert's Organics (www.albertsorganics.com) carries an enormous inventory of organic meat and other food products.

Lamb is a great choice, as it is often less expensive than beef and is usually grass fed, especially when from New Zealand.

MEAT SUBSTITUTES

As mentioned, I suggest eating unfermented soy as a meat substitute very sparingly. Instead look for tempeh and seitan, which are delicious and extremely nutritious. I love these:

West Soy Seitan and West Soy Chicken-Style Seitan (www.westsoy.biz) are available at many grocery and health food stores.

Lightlife Tempeh (www.lightlife.com) is available at most large health food stores.

STOCKS AND BROTHS

I mention the use of stocks in many of my recipes. It's always best to make your own, but if you can't, look for the following brands:

Pacific Foods organic broths (www.pacificfoods.com)

Imagine organic broths (www.imaginefoods.com)

Trader Joe's organic broths

These boxes can get pricey, so it's a good idea to use bouillon cubes instead. Make sure that the cubes you choose are free of MSG and other nasty additives—I like:

Organic Gourmet Vegetable Bouillon Cubes (www.selectfreshcuisine.com)
Rapunzel Vegan Vegetable Bouillon Cubes (www.veganessentials.com)
Organic Harvest Sun Bouillon Cubes (www.theveganstore.com)

FISH

All your fish needs to be from a sustainable source, so don't forget to look for the "MSC-Certified label," or log on to www.mbayaq.org to get the skinny on any fish that you are thinking of buying.

The best low-mercury tunas are:

Wild Planet (www.wildplanet.com)
American Tuna (www.americantuna.com)

It costs three times as much as regular tuna, so eat it twice a month instead of twice a week. The tuna have been extensively tested by independent labs and have a minimal amount of mercury.

Canned salmon is less costly and a great alternative.

365 Pink Wild Salmon (Whole Foods)
Pure Alaska Salmon Company (www.purealaskasalmon.com)

EGGS

Many large grocery chains now carry their own line of organic eggs for a decent price. Also check out www.organicvalley.coop to see if you can get a coupon or two!

Remember that the only label that is meaningful on an egg carton is "organic"— so don't waste your time and money on any other claims, such as "cage-free" or "fertile." Organic eggs cost considerably more, but you are getting what you pay for, so it's best to eat eggs twice a week instead of every day and treat yourself to the best.

I recommend the following brands in stores:

Organic Valley
Trader Joe's organic
Whole Foods 365 Organic
Kroger Private Selection Organic

FLOURS AND GRAINS

For delicious yellow corn grits, I love Arrowhead Mills organic yellow corn grits (www.arrowheadmills.com). Most large chain grocery stores carry their own store-brand organic flours.

BREAD

SPROUTED-GRAIN BREADS

My favorite is called Ezekiel 4:9 by Food for Life (www.foodforlife.com). It's available in many of the major grocery stores and in virtually every health food store. They also make sprouted-grain tortillas, muffins, cereals, and pastas.

Alvarado Street Bakery (www.alvaradostreetbakery.com) also has a great line of sprouted-grain breads.

Sprouted grains are also made into manna bread, and, boy, is this delicious! It's dense and chewy and is absolutely heavenly toasted and spread with butter or ghee. Find the most delectable manna bread at www.naturespath.com.

When buying whole-wheat breads, make sure the label says "100% whole wheat" on it and that there is no high-fructose corn syrup in the ingredient list.

Most of the large grocery chains now have their own organic brand breads.

I also recommend:

Arnold 100% Whole Wheat bread
Oroweat 100% Whole Wheat bread

If you have a bread maker, be sure to buy organic whole-wheat bread flour. I actually love using bread mixes when I'm short of time—here are two great brands:

Barry Farm (www.barryfarm.com) has a great selection of bread mixes and
    I love them all.
Pepper Creek Farm (www.worldpantry.com) has a fabulous bread mix sampler, which is great for testing out on your friends and family!
Purcell Mountain Farms (www.purcellmountainfarms.com)

BREAKFAST CEREALS

I have suggested throughout most of the eating plan that you either make your own granola or use steel-cut or old-fashioned oats. All these ingredients are available (organic) in your local health food store. Try to buy from bulk bins and you will save a lot and not have an extra cardboard box to recycle.

I have suggested the following cereals and granolas, as either breakfasts for the on-the-go girl or snacks.

Kashi cereals are an excellent choice because they use a variety of whole grains. I like the Whole Grain Puffs and the Kashi GoLean. These are available at most large grocery chains.

I recommend Nature's Path (www.naturespath.com) Organic Hemp Plus Granola. My daughter loves it because it's sweet and nutty, and I like it because it contains a lot of omega-3 fatty acids from the hemp. It's available in most large grocery chains.

Galaxy Granola (www.galaxygranola.com) is organic and makes the yummiest snack on earth. It's sold in a wide selection of grocery and health food stores.

Cascadian Farm (www.cascadianfarm.com) has a a great selection of organic cereals.

CRACKERS AND CHIPS

Crackers can contain so many undesirable additives that you need to be really careful with your label reading. I recommend the following, which are available in many grocery and health food store chains:

Ry Krisp
Finn Crisp
Late July Organic Crackers
Kavli Flat Breads
Mary's Gone Crackers
Ak-Mak Whole of the Wheat Crackers
Kashi TLC crackers

Doctor Kracker
Lundberg Original Sea Salt Rice Chips

COCONUT OIL AND BUTTER

I recommend using unrefined virgin coconut oil, since the refining process involves chemicals and bleaching agents.

In grocery stores, you will find Spectrum's organic virgin unrefined coconut oil.

Tropical Traditions (www.tropicaltraditions.com) carries some of the best-quality coconut products available.

You will also find a great coconut oil at Nutiva (www.nutiva.com).

My biggest treat is a spoonful of raw coconut butter made by Artisana (www.premierorganics.com). A large jar will last you a long time and just a teaspoon straight or in a smoothie will fill you up and keep you really healthy. You can also freeze it and make divinely healthy popsicles.

CANNED AND FROZEN VEGETABLES

I am really careful about buying canned fruits and veggies because of the BPA-leaching issue. This is a class of hormone-disrupting chemicals that are often found in the lining of cans. If you are really keen on a particular brand, I suggest you call or e-mail the company to find out whether or not they still use this chemical.

The only foods I recommend buying in cans are tomatoes (in the winter) and beans. The only company that I can fully recommend at the time of printing is Eden Foods. They have an excellent green history and philosophy in every respect and their foods are of the highest quality. I think their canned beans are the best and I use them frequently because I can't always be bothered with the soaking thing; and I love that they absolutely do not use any leaching can liners whatsoever.

Eden Foods (www.edenfoods.com) sells a wide variety of beans and tomatoes and *does not* use bisphenol A in the can linings.

In the winter, I often buy frozen berries, peas, corn, and green beans.

Whole Foods has its own 365 brand.

I also like Cascadian Farm (www.cascadianfarm.com), which is available at many large grocery and health food stores.

CONDIMENTS

MAYONNAISE AND OTHER DRESSINGS

Since dressings are so easy to make, I recommend that you never buy bottled ones from the store—most of them are filled with preservatives, flavor enhancers, thickeners, and so on. If you're feeling lazy, just dress your salad with extra-virgin olive oil and lemon juice.

Homemade mayonnaise is a little more complicated, so here are the store brands I suggest:

Spectrum Organic Mayonnaise (www.spectrumorganics.com)
Hain's Safflower mayonnaise

Note: Many of the vegan mayo spreads are likely to contain high-fructose corn syrup, so read your ingredient list.

SAUCES, MUSTARDS, ETC.

I like to buy my ketchup in a glass bottle because it's easier to recycle.

Tropical Traditions carries a wonderful ketchup, which is sweetened with agave (www.tropicaltraditions.com).

If you like Worcestershire sauce, you get can a great vegan one called the Wizard's Vegan Worcestershire Sauce (www.edwardandsons.com).

I love Busha Browne (www.bushabrowne.com) Planter's Steak Sauce—yum! It's vegan and works well with meat, tempeh, veggies, and just about anything.

My favorite mustards are:

Westbrae Natural
365 Organic Mustard (Whole Foods)
Grey Poupon

SALT

It's really important that you purchase unrefined sea salt as opposed to plain sea salt—this is because the refining process strips the salt of all its valuable minerals and adds many agents, including bleaching agents to bring you the white stuff!

If you like salt, as I do, invest in the best:

Le Tresor Organic Sea Salt (www.ezoetic.com)
SaltWorks Sea Salt (www.webvitamins.com)

Remember, salt is salt as far as blood pressure goes, so go easy!

COOKIES AND TREATS

The following treats are my favorites and can be found at many large grocery stores:

Zen Bakery Blueberry Fiber Cakes (Trader Joe's and Whole Foods)
Andean Dream Quinoa Cookies (www.andeanquinoa.com)
The GoodOnYa bar (www.thegoodonyabar.com): These are so good, it's
    worth ordering a box.
Lundberg Rice Cakes, honey nut (www.lundberg.com)
True North Almond Clusters (www.truenorthnuts.com)
Theo Chocolate (www.theochocolate.com)
Purely Decadent Coconut Craze Soy Ice Cream (www.purelydecadent
    .com)

NUTS

Make sure all the nuts you buy are raw (not roasted or salted)
    I buy almost all of my nuts from Trader Joe's because they have a great selection
and are relatively inexpensive or come in bulk bins.
    Share a delivery from www.bulkfoods.com with a friend.

TEAS AND COFFEES

Many large grocery stores and coffee shops now carry organic and/or fair-trade coffees. Also look out for store brands, which are less expensive.

Good Earth Coffee (www.goodearthcoffee.com) is organic, is inexpensive,
    has green packaging, and is widely available.
Teeccino (www.teeccino.com) is a fantastic coffee substitute. It is creamy
    and nutty and comes in all sorts of different flavors.

I am a passionate tea drinker. I love the taste and also the fact that most green teas (my favorite) have a fraction of the amount of caffeine that coffee has. Here are some great companies:

Yogi Tea (www.yogitea.com)
Rishi Tea (www.rishi-tea.com)
Eden Foods (www.edenfoods.com)
Numi Tea (www.numitea.com)
Strand Tea (www.strandtea.com)
The organic teas at Celestial Seasonings (www.celestialseasonings.com)
DōMatcha (www.domatcha.com)

TEA AND COFFEE ACCESSORIES

I love the Wisdom Wand (www.wisdomwands.com). It's a glass straw with a filter on the end, which stops your teeth from becoming stained. You can get the one with a filter for tea or one for coffee.

I also love the Tea Tiger from Strand Teas (www.strandtea.com). It's a beautiful tea mug with a filter, so you can brew your tea (and watch it brew, since it's clear) on the run.

SWEETENERS

HONEY

I always recommend buying raw honey. Make sure that the label actually says "Raw," not "Unheated."

MAPLE SYRUP

It's really important to buy organic maple syrup because nonorganic syrups use formaldehyde in the extraction process. Grade B is less expensive and contains a good amount of nutrients.

I love using maple sugar as a sweetener because it is packed with nutrients and isn't as sweetie-sweet as sugar. You can order it online from www.maplesource.com.

STEVIA

You can now buy stevia at most grocery stores. However, I like to use the green powder stevia, which contains more nutrients.

You can buy Health & Herbs Stevia (Green) Powder at www.herbalremedies.com.

SUPPLEMENTS

You'll find a really comprehensive selection of supplements for women at New Chapter (www.newchapter.com). I use their Estrotone supplement to relieve PMS symptoms. This company also has an organic farm and is committed to protecting the environment.

Fish oils (www.nordicnaturals.com)
Hemp seed oil (www.nutiva.com)
Vitamins for women (www.realfoodorganics.com)
Green Superfoods:
Balance by Cosmedix (www.cosmedix.com)
Pure Synergy (www.synergy-co.com)

KITCHEN APPLIANCES

BREAD MAKERS

The common complaint with bread makers is that the Teflon coating can peel off or be harmful when brought to a high temperature. I recommend the Zojuirushi BBCC-X20 or the miniversion because the nonstick coating doesn't peel off at all. It also makes excellent bread.

YOGURT MAKERS

I love the Cuisipro Donvier Electronic Yogurt Maker. It comes with small glass containers. You can order at either www.amazon.com or www.thekitchenstore.com.

I also like the Yogourmet. It comes with a plastic jar, so I recommend that you order the spare glass jar and use it instead. This model works if you are space challenged. You can buy it with all the necessary powder cultures from www.lucyskitchenshop.com.

SODA MAKER

Soda Stream (www.sodaclubusa.com) is the greenest appliance you can buy because it avoids so much packaging and it'll save you a lot of money, too.

POTS AND PANS

I recommend Cuisinart's Green Gourmet hard anodized collection (www.cuisinart .com).

I recommend all of Chantal's high-quality cookware, especially the copper-fusion line (www.chantal.com).

I love preseasoned cast-iron skillets and the enamel Dutch ovens from Lodge (www.lodgemfg.com).

Chantal's new Pure line of dye-free bakeware is a fantastic eco-friendly line that is microwave oven and dishwasher safe.

UTENSILS

Chantal (www.chantal.com) carries the most exquisite stainless steel utensils ever. I haven't found a better garlic crusher, and I feel it's worth the investment since I crush garlic almost every day.

CUTTING BOARDS, COLANDERS, ETC.

I love bamboo cutting boards. Totally Bamboo (www.totallybamboo.com) has created the GreenLite cutting board, which is featherlight, durable, and dishwasher safe. This company is dedicated to sustainable and eco-conscious practices.

I make sure that I get all my picnicware and more from www.recycline.com. They carry fabulous colanders, reusable flatware, and fantastic screw-top storage containers. They partner with the yogurt company Stonyfield Farm, and everything is made from recycled yogurt cups.

PAPER PRODUCTS

Make sure that all your paper products are made from 100-percent recycled paper. This includes kitchen towels, napkins, and toilet paper.

The following brands, which are available at many large grocery chains and big box stores, are made from 100-percent recycled paper:

365 at Whole Foods

Best Value

Atlantic

Earth First

Fiesta

Green Forest

Marcal

Planet

Seventh Generation

Trader Joe's paper towels and toilet paper are made from postconsumer content.

ECO-FRIENDLY NONTOXIC CLEANING SUPPLIES

I love the Method products (www.methodhome.com) for my kitchen. They are in cool-looking containers and are really effective.

I particularly like:

Smarty Dish for your dishwasher

Steel for Real for your stainless

Daily Granite for your granite surfaces

Wood for Good for your wood

I also love a company called BioKleen (www.biokleenhome.com).

I particularly like:

Hand Moisturizing Dishwashing Liquid

Free and Clear Automatic Dishwashing Powder

ECO-FRIENDLY KITCHEN SUPPLIES

Instead of plastic bags to store produce, I use bamboo cloth bags, which keep everything, even bread, fresh for days. Order from www.bamboo-bag.com. I also like organic cotton produce bags from www.bluelotusblankets.com. For more eco-friendly trash bags, check out www.perfgogreen.com and www.greenlinepaper.com.

GARDENING

OUTDOOR

My favorite composter is:

The Garden Gourmet (www.gardengourmet.com).

You can buy composting enzymes and a special turner (a pitchfork will work as well) from www.realgoods.com.

To buy a worm bin and the worms, visit Uncle Jim at www.unclejimswormfarm .com.

For a great selection of rain barrels, including the "eco-barrel," go to www .greenculture.com.

For a beautiful wooden raised garden bed, go to www.greenculture.com.

For heirloom seeds, visit www.heirloomseeds.com and consider their Victory Garden Package. For every one of these purchased, they will donate $10 to the American Red Cross. The package includes a huge variety of great edible plants.

A great seeds resource is www.seedsofchange.com.

For garden pests, the Cook's Garden (www.cooksgarden.com) has a good selection of nontoxic repellents.

INDOOR

For compost crocks visit www.gorgeouslygreen.com/catalog.

A fantastic indoor compost system called the Sakura Kitchen Compost Bin is available at www.greenculture.com.

If you live in a cool northern climate and want to grow herbs and salads in the winter, consider the Aerogrow planter (www.aerogrow.com).

EXERCISE AND FITNESS

For the best eco-friendly yoga mats, go to www.turninglife.com.

You can also go here to buy the Eco Exercise Body Toning Kit, which includes a ball and bands for an arm and thigh workout.

For a great rebounder that folds up under your bed, go to www.needak-rebounders.com.

The best home yoga DVDs are by the brilliant teacher Natasha Rizopoulos (www.natasharizopoulos.com). She is a fantastic instructor for both beginners and more seasoned yogis. She makes yoga simple and easy to understand.

My favorite home fitness DVDs are:

The Bar Method (www.barmethod.com)
Zumba (www.zumba.com)

Buy beautiful organic sports and yoga clothes at:

www.bluecanoe.com
www.prana.com
www.patagonia.com

For eco-friendly running shoes, New Balance (www.newbalance.com) is a good choice. They are one of the most socially responsible companies in their field. They have phased out the toxic PVC from all their products.

Also check out the Cascadia shoe at www.brooksrunning.com.

Save up for a pair of MBT sports shoes (www.swissmasaius.com); they will work your legs and correct your posture while walking, working out, or just standing in line!

USEFUL CHART: WHERE DO YOU BUY IT?

	REGULAR GROCERY STORE	WEB SITE	HEALTH FOOD GROCERY STORE
Dairy			
Straus Family Farms Dairy Products www.strausfamily creamery.com		X	
Stonyfield Farms Yogurts www.stonyfieldfarm .com	X	X	
Rachel's Yogurts www.rachelsdairy .com		X	

(Continued)

(Continued)

	REGULAR GROCERY STORE	WEB SITE	HEALTH FOOD GROCERY STORE
Lifeway Kefir www.lifeway.net	X	X	
Oikos Yogurt www.oikosyogurt.com		X	
Fage Yogurt www.fageusa.com	X	X	
Organic Valley Dairy Products www.organicvalley .coop/		X	
Kerrygold Butter www.kerrygold.com	X	X	
Soy/Dairy Alternatives			
West Soy Seitan www.westsoy.biz		X	
Lightlife Tempeh www.lightlife.com		X	
Soya Kaas Soy Cheese	X		
Lisanatti Cheese www.lisanatticheese .com		X	
Meat/Fish			
Niman Ranch www.nimanranch .com		X	X
Applegate Farms www.applegatefarms .com		X	X
Wild Harvest Organic www.wildharvest organic.com	X	X	
Petaluma Poultry www.petalumapoultry .com		X	X

(Continued)

(Continued)

	REGULAR GROCERY STORE	WEB SITE	HEALTH FOOD GROCERY STORE
American Tuna www.americantuna .com		X	X
Wild Planet Tuna www.1wildplanet.com		X	X
Breads/Crackers/ Cereals			
Arrowhead Mills Oatmeal www.arrowheadmills .com		X	X
Bob's Red Mill Scottish Oatmeal www.bobsredmill.com		X	X
Peace Cereal www.peacecereal.com		X	X
Galaxy Granola www.galaxygranola .com	X	X	X
Dylan's Chia Granola www.dylanschia.com		X	X
Nature's Path Cereals and Oatmeal www.naturespath.com	X	X	X
Food for Life Sprouted Grain Bread www.foodforlife.com		X	
Alvarado Street Spouted Grain www.alvaradostreet bakery.com		X	
Nature's Path Manna Bread www.naturespath.com		X	
Ry Krisp Crackers www.bremnerfood group.com	X	X	

(Continued)

(Continued)

	Regular Grocery Store	Web Site	Health Food Grocery Store
Finn Crisp Crackers	X		
Late July Crackers www.latejuly.com		X	X
Kavli Flat Breads	X		
Mary's Gone Crackers www.marys gonecrackers.com		X	X
Doctor Kracker www.drkracker.com		X	X
Kashi TLC www.kashi.com	X	X	
Ak-Mak crackers www.akmakbakeries .com	X	X	
Lundberg Rice Chips www.lundberg.com		X	X
Pasta/Rice/Beans			
Deboles Pasta www.deboles.com		X	X
Ancient Harvest Pasta www.quinoa.net		X	X
Eden Pasta www.edenfoods.com		X	X
Condiments/Oils			
Spectrum Cooking oils www.spectrumorganics .com	X	X	X
Nutiva Virgin Coconut and hemp products www.nutiva.com		X	X
Virgin Coconut oil www.tropical traditions.com		X	X

(Continued)

(*Continued*)

	REGULAR GROCERY STORE	WEB SITE	HEALTH FOOD GROCERY STORE
Eden Organic Olive oil www.edenfoods.com		X	X
Figueroa Farms Organic Olive Oil www.figueroafarms .com		X	X
Wilderness Family Naturals Coconut Products www.wilderness familynaturals.com		X	X
Spectrum Mayo www.spectrum organics.com	X	X	X
Hains Safflower Mayo www.hainspurefoods .com	X	X	
Follow Your Heart Vegan Mayo www .followyourheart.com		X	
Wizard's Organic Worcestershire Sauce www.edwardandsons .com		X	X
Busha Browne's Planter's Steak Sauce			X
Westbrae Natural's Organic mustard www.westbrae.com	X	X	X
Protein Bars/ Powders			
Jay Robb bars and powders www.jayrobb.com		X	X

(*Continued*)

(Continued)

	Regular Grocery Store	Web Site	Health Food Grocery Store
Whey Protein Greens Plus www.greensplus.com	X	X	X
Think Organic/Think Green www.think products.com		X	X
Larabar www.larabar.com	X	X	X
Sweets and Treats			
Sweet Dreams Brown Rice Syrup www.lundberg.com		X	X
Purely Decadent Coconut Craze Ice-Cream www.purelydecadent .com		X	
Theo Chocolate www.theochocolate .com		X	X
Sjaaks Chocolate www.sjaaks.com		X	X
Dagoba Chocolate www.dagobachocolate .com		X	X
Zen Bakery Fiber Cakes www.zenbakery.com	X	X	
Andean Dream Cookies www.andeandream .com		X	X
Dr. Oetker's Cake Mix www.oetker.us	X	X	X

(Continued)

354 - THE *Gorgeously* GREEN DIET

	REGULAR GROCERY STORE	WEB SITE	HEALTH FOOD GROCERY STORE
Tea/Coffee			
Good Earth Coffee www.goodearthcoffee.com	X	X	X
Equal Exchange Coffee www.equalexchange.coop	X	X	X
Yogi Tea www.yogitea.com	X	X	X
Mountain Rose Herb Bulk Teas			X
DōMatcha Tea www.domatcha.com		X	X
Strand Tea www.strandtea.com		X	
Miscellaneous			
Pacific Foods Organic Broth		X	X
Imagine Organic Broth www.imaginefoods.com	X	X	X
Organic Harvest Sun Bouillon Cubes			X
Organic Gourmet Vegetable Bouillon Cubes www.organic-gourmet.com	X	X	
Rapunzel Vegan Bouillon Cubes www.rapunzel.com		X	X
Eden Canned Tomatoes and all kind of beans www.edenfoods.com		X	X

(Continued)

	Regular Grocery Store	Web Site	Health Food Grocery Store
Amy's Organic Veggie Burgers and frozen food www.amyskitchen.com	X	X	
Cascadian Farms Organic Frozen Vegetables www.cascadianfarm .com	X	X	
Pacific Foods Nut Milks www.pacificfoods.com	X	X	X
Manitoba Harvest Hemp Milk www.manitobaharvest .com		X	X
Dried Apricots www.apricotking.com		X	X
Macadamia nuts www.livingtree community.com		X	X
Beverages			
Odwalla Super–Protein Smoothie www.odwalla.com	X	X	
Walnut Acres Juices www.walnutacres.com	X	X	X

RECOMMENDED READING

Animal, Vegetable, Miracle by Barbara Kingsolver

Blessed Unrest by Paul Hawken

The Coconut Oil Miracle by Bruce Fife, CN, ND

The Whole Soy Story: The Dark Side of America's Favorite Health Food by Kaayla T. Daniel, PhD, CNN

The Detox Solution by Patricia Fitzgerald

Eat Fat Lose Fat by Dr. Mary Enig and Sally Fallon

The End of Food by Paul Roberts

How to Grow More Vegetables by John Jeavons

In Defense of Food by Michael Pollan

The Omnivore's Dilemma by Michael Pollan

The Organic Cook's Bible by Jeff Cox

Plenty by Alisa Smith and J. B. Mackinnon

The Stolen Harvest by Vandana Shiva

For a complete bibliography, visit www.gorgeouslygreen.com/bibliography

RECOMMENDED WEB SITES

www.jhsph.edu

www.foodandwaterwatch.org

www.nrdc.org

www.bornfreeusa.org

www.ewg.org

ACKNOWLEDGMENTS

A handful of extraordinary people helped to make this book possible and I am so incredibly grateful to them.

First and foremost, I want to thank my partner in crime and love of my life, Joe. Your support and unwavering patience have not only made this journey possible, but also made it a blast. You are a part of every page of this book.

To my little muse, Lola. You inspire me to pass on everything that my mother has passed on to me about the joy of exquisite food.

To my beautiful mother, who taught me that one of the greatest delights in life is cooking and eating. You showed me that nourishing family and friends with real food, the best that you could find, is a truly spiritual experience.

I thank my father, who taught me that a successful diet should simply be one that allows pretty much *everything,* in moderation. Your passion for good food is infectious.

I am so thankful to the entire Uliano family: Dalio, Bobbie, Kay, and Dan— your unyielding support of the Gorgeously Green message has been invaluable. A special thank you to Kay for stepping up to the plate and being my guinea pig in all things Gorgeously Green.

To Amy Hertz, my brilliant editor, whose expert guidance and humor have been paramount in this adventure.

A big thanks to all at Dutton who worked so hard to make this book as beautiful and coherent as it is. A special thank you to Melissa Miller.

Scott Waxman, my agent, who understood where I was trying to go, even before I did! Thank you for your wise direction, which always lands me in the right place.

Heartfelt praise and gratitude go to Dr. Julia Tatum-Hunter, who has made such an incredibly valuable contribution to this book. Thank you for your knowledge, expertise, and deep, intuitive wisdom.

Marcus and Jane Buckingham, who continue to be a source of great inspiration. Jane, you are an angel, and Marcus, a mentor. I cannot thank you both enough for giving me so much of your precious time.

Marcy Engelman, my publicist, who is simply the very best.

Thank you, Emily Hart, for your beautiful photographs, your generosity, and your bright spirit.

I want to acknowledge all the women in my life who make my writing possible when the going gets rough, especially Kim Swann, whom I have been able to rely on many times to take care of my precious one.

Thank you also to a group of women who have helped and inspired me along the way: Colleen Vinetz, Mary Lyn Rapier, Cami Taylor, Julie Mollo, and Martha Chang.

Finally I want to acknowledge all the incredible women who have joined the Gorgeously Green community and shared with me your stories of transformation. You are the change and there is nothing more important.

INDEX